4th Edition

RNotes®

Nurse's Clinical Pocket Guide

Ehren Myers, RN

Purchase additional copies of this book at your health science bookstore or directly from F.A. Davis by shopping online at www.fadavis.com or by calling 800-323-3555 (US) or 800-665-1148 (CAN)

A Davis's Notes Book

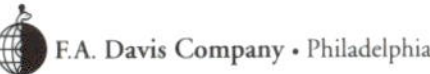
F.A. Davis Company • Philadelphia

1915 Arch Street
Philadelphia, PA 19103
www.fadavis.com

Printed in China by Imago

Last digit indicates print number: 10 9 8 7 6 5 4 3 2 1

Publisher, Nursing: Robert G. Martone
Director of Content Development: Darlene D. Pedersen
Content Project Manager: Victoria White
Design & Illustrations Manager: Carolyn O'Brien
Reviewers: For a complete list of reviewers, go to davisplus.fadavis.com, and enter keyword "Myers."

Place 2⅞ × 2⅞ **Sticky Notes** here
for a convenient and refillable note pad

✓**HIPAA Compliant**
✓**OSHA Compliant**

Waterproof and Reusable Wipe-Free Pages

Write directly onto any page of *RNotes* with a ballpoint pen. Wipe old entries off with an alcohol pad and reuse.

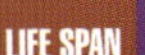

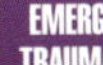

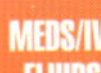

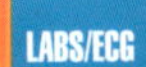

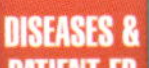

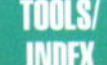

PRE-PROCEDURE GUIDELINES

- Confirm that the order (if needed) is in Pt's chart and ensure that a signed consent is present (if required).
- Review medical record for allergies and conditions that may influence Pt's ability to tolerate procedure.
- Observe the "6 Rights of Medication Administration" when giving medications, and triple-check all medication orders.
- Gather and assemble necessary supplies, and obtain assistance from additional staff as needed.
- Perform hand hygiene before contact with Pt, before and after putting on gloves, and before exiting Pt's room.
- Use standard precautions during every Pt contact.
- Prepare the Pt; explain the procedure and offer reassurance.
- Identify the Pt; use a minimum of 2 identifiers (e.g., name and date of birth) and compare against information on Pt's chart and ID band. Use verbal confirmation when possible.
- Ensure there is proper lighting (rooms are often dark).
- Adjust bed height (usually to level of your elbows) and lower nearest side rail to facilitate proper body mechanics.
- Provide comfort and maintain privacy, exposing only what is minimally necessary to perform procedure.

POST-PROCEDURE GUIDELINES

- Discard soiled items and sharps into appropriate containers.
- Follow institutional policy regarding recyclable items.
- Clean and store (or remove) reusable equipment.
- Discard gloves and wash hands before touching or handling unsoiled items (e.g., side rails, personal items).
- Clean and dry the Pt and replace linens as necessary.
- Return the Pt to a position of comfort.
- Raise side rails and lower bed to lowest position.
- Ensure tubes and lines are free of kinks and obstruction.
- Ensure call light and Pt items are within easy reach.
- Document procedure, Pt's response, and assessment findings.
- **Medication:** Document dose, route, time, site, and Pt's response.

Head-tilt, Chin-lift

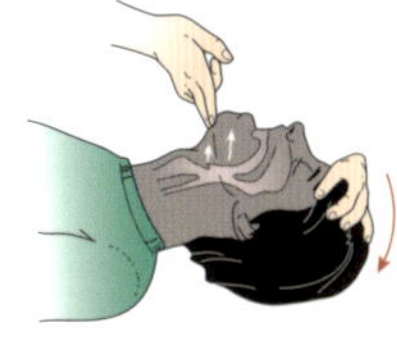

1. Push down gently on Pt's forehead.
2. Pull up on bony part of chin with 2–3 fingers of your dominant hand.
3. Make sure line from chin to jaw angle is perpendicular to floor; head and neck should be slightly extended; an infant's head should be in a neutral position (sniffing position).
4. Lift mandible upward and outward.
5. Avoid obstructing airway by closing mouth or compressing chin soft tissue.

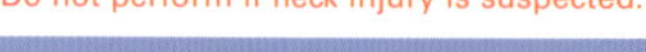

Do not perform if neck injury is suspected.

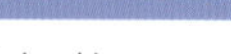

Jaw-thrust

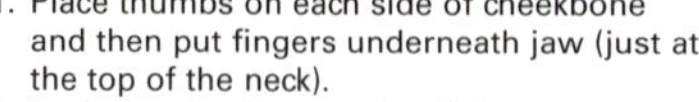

1. Place thumbs on each side of cheekbone and then put fingers underneath jaw (just at the top of the neck).
2. Push thumbs down and pull fingers up.
3. Hold this position so tongue will not fall back into throat, blocking airway.

Recommended for Pts with a suspected neck injury.

Airway—Nasal and Oral

Nasopharyngeal Airway (NPA)

Use for Breathing Pts With a Gag Reflex

1. Measure from tip of Pt's nose to earlobe, and select a tube with a diameter about the size of the Pt's smallest finger.
2. Lubricate the tube with water-soluble lubricant, and insert with bevel toward septum using the measured length of tube.
3. Right nostril: Insert straight back until flange rests against nostril.
4. Left nostril: Insert straight back and then rotate 180° once you reach the posterior pharynx.

NASOPHARYNGEAL AIRWAY

PHARYNX
NASOPHARYNGEAL AIRWAY
TRACHEA
ESOPHAGUS

◎ Never use in presence of facial or head trauma.

Oropharyngeal Airway (OPA)

Use for Unconscious Pts Without a Gag Reflex

1. Measure from corner of Pt's mouth to earlobe.
   - **Adults and larger children**: Insert OPA upside down and rotate 180° as it passes back of tongue, past soft palette, until flange rests on Pt's lips.
   - **Small children**: Using tongue depressor, insert OPA right side up along normal curve of oral cavity until flange rests on Pt's lips.

OROPHARYNGEAL AIRWAY

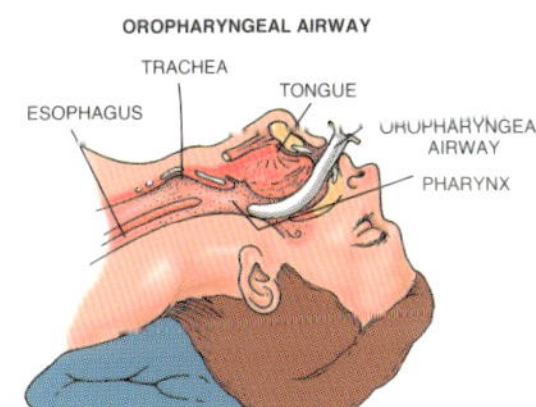

Elastic Stockings (TED Hose)

Thigh-high: Measure each leg from gluteal fold to base of heel. Measure each calf circumference and thigh at widest parts. If both legs do not measure the same size, obtain 2 different sized stockings, using one from each package to make 2 pairs.

Knee-high: Measure from base of heel to middle of knee joint and record circumference of calf at the widest point.

Procedure

1. Position and instruct Pt to remain supine for 15 min or elevate feet and legs as tolerated for 15 min.
2. Cleanse legs and feet as needed and thoroughly dry; follow manufacturer's recommendation on use of talcum powder.
3. Hold stocking by cuff in dominant hand, slide nondominant hand into stocking to the heel, grasp heel with hand inside stocking, then turn stocking inside out to level of heel.
4. Instruct Pt to keep toes pointed and gently ease stocking onto foot, centering Pt's heel in heel of stocking.
5. Pull remainder of stocking up and over leg, turning it right side out, to gluteal fold for thigh-high stockings or 1–2 in. below knee for knee-high stockings.
6. Ensure stocking is straight and free of wrinkles to minimize risk of skin breakdown and constricted circulation.
7. If using a closed-toe stocking, pull gently on end of stocking over toe to create a small space in front of toes.
8. Assess every shift (or as ordered) for skin color, temperature, sensation, movement, and swelling, and remove once per shift (or as ordered) for 20–30 min.

Apical-Radial Pulse

1. Positioning: HOB elevated to level of comfort.
2. Obtain assistance from second nurse—the first nurse to palpate radial pulse and the second nurse to auscultate apical pulse simultaneously.
3. Expose left chest and locate cardiac apex by palpating the fifth intercostal space along the left midclavicular line.
4. Designate one nurse to observe watch, stating "Start" and then "Stop" after 60 sec.
5. Start counting pulses simultaneously when nurse observing watch says, "Start."
6. Count pulses for 60 sec.
7. Stop counting and record measurements when designated nurse says, "Stop."
8. Compare and record results.

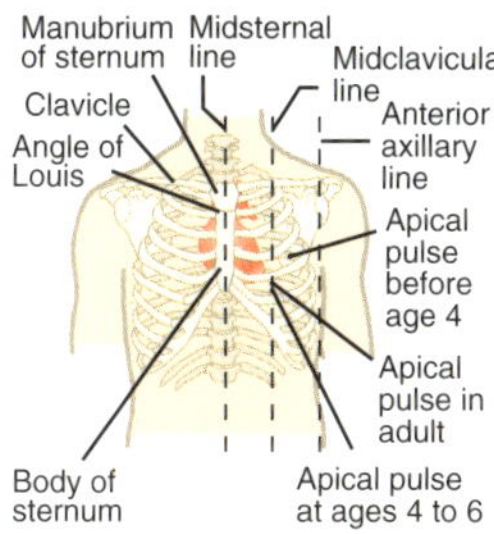

Assess for Apical-Radial Pulse Deficit

Apical-Radial Pulse Deficit (if present)

- Subtract radial pulse from apical pulse.
- The difference is the apical-radial pulse deficit.
- Report an apical-radial pulse deficit to the HCP.

Pts with pulse deficits must be assessed for additional signs of decreased cardiac output such as variations in BP, tachycardia, restlessness, and change in mental status.

Aspiration Precautions

General Guidelines

1. Positioning: 90° upright during meals; instruct Pt to remain upright for 30–60 min after meals; never rush Pt.
2. Assess Pt for dysphagia/aspiration risk using institution-specific screening tool and enter in Pt's chart.
3. Observe Pt for drooling, coughing, gagging, and choking—have suction available and suction airway as needed.
4. Inspect Pt's mouth for pocketing of food.
5. Instruct Pt to use a chin-to-chest posture during initial assessment—begin with small sips of water and progress to larger volumes and different consistencies.
6. Use thickener for thin liquids—follow packaging directions.
7. Place food on unaffected side in Pts with hemiparesis.
8. Monitor Pt's weight weekly.

Signs of Dysphagia

- Weakness or poor muscle tone of neck, lips, face, or tongue
- Poor posture or head control
- Drooling or difficulty managing secretions
- Poor oral hygiene (e.g., thrush)
- Confusion, dementia, or stroke
- Slurred or difficult speech or wet voice after eating
- Cough—during meals or shortly after swallowing
- Generalized weakness or fatigues easily during meals

Assistive Devices

- Pt may be unsteady—be prepared to catch Pt.
- Use a gait belt and obtain extra staff as needed.

Canes

1. Position cane on unaffected (stronger) side approximately 6 in. (or closer) laterally to side of foot.
2. Elbow should be flexed at a comfortable angle.
3. Support weight with cane—repeat the following steps:
4. Advance cane forward to a comfortable distance (~12 in.).
5. Advance weaker leg so that it is parallel to the cane.
6. Advance stronger leg beyond the cane to a comfortable distance (heel just beyond the cane).
7. Advance weaker leg until it is parallel to the stronger leg.

Crutches

1. Position crutch tips 6 in. laterally and 6 in. in front of Pt's feet—adjust per Pt comfort level.
2. Adjust crutch height to accommodate 2–3 finger widths between crutch pad and axillae.
3. Elbows should be slightly flexed when resting palms on hand grips—Pt should never bear weight on axillary pads.
4. Support weight with crutches—repeat the following steps:
5. Advance both crutches and weaker leg to a comfortable distance (~12 in.), supporting weight with hands
6. Advance stronger leg until it is parallel with crutches.

Walkers—Avoid Using on Stairs

1. Position walker so that Pt can stand comfortably upright while holding hand grips; elbows should be slightly flexed.
2. Support weight with walker—repeat the following steps:
3. Instruct Pt to move walker forward 6 in.
4. Ensure that all 4 legs are firmly on ground.
5. Step forward using walker for balance and stability.

Bladder Irrigation, Continuous (CBI)

Setup

1. Hang irrigation bag on IV pole.
2. Connect and prime irrigation tubing to bag.
3. Cleanse irrigation port of triple-lumen urinary catheter and attach irrigation tubing.
4. Ensure drainage port from catheter is patent.

Procedure

1. Begin irrigation at prescribed rate.
2. Monitor drainage output for the following:
   - Color and clarity—normal is pink and free of clots (notify HCP if red or has clots)
   - Blood clots, sediment, or kinks in tubing
   - Decreased or no output (drainage output should be greater than irrigation input)
3. Monitor Pt for bladder distention, spasm, or pain.
4. Calculate urine output by subtracting total volume of irrigant infused from total volume of fluid collected in drainage bag.
5. Document findings.

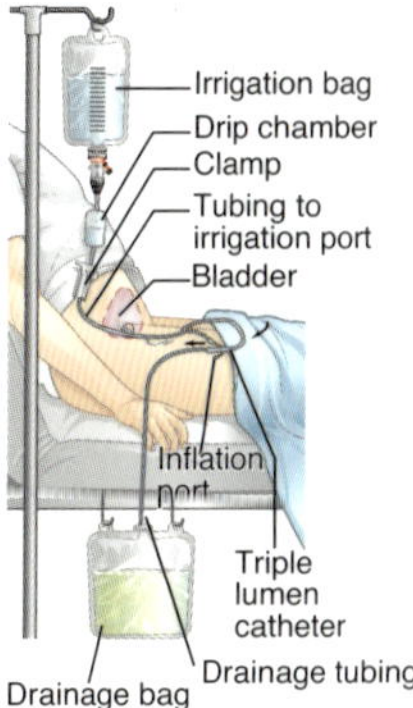

Bladder Scanner

Indications

Assessment of: Bladder volume; urinary retention; post-void residual volume.

Procedure

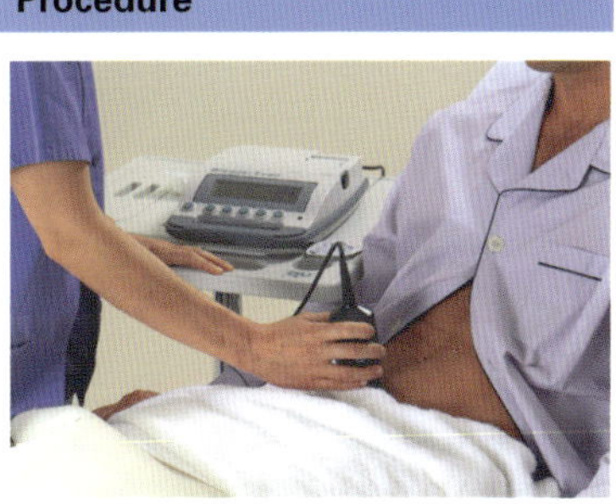

1. Positioning: Supine; HOB may be elevated for comfort.
2. Select sex on bladder scanner.
3. Select "male" for women with hysterectomy.
4. Apply ultrasound transmission gel to probe head.
5. Position scanning probe midline, 1 in. above symphysis pubis (pointed at bladder).
6. Do not move probe head during scan.
7. Record volume and notify HCP as indicated.

◎ Contraindicated during pregnancy or if a wound is present in the area to be scanned.

◎ Volumes less than 250 mL usually will not induce urinary urge.

Blood Administration

For Transfusion Reaction, see EMERG/TRAUMA.

Supplies

- IV start kit
- 0.9% saline solution
- Informed consent
- Blood bank armband and administration form
- Blood administration tubing with inline filter
- A separate line for fluid and medications
- An 18-gauge catheter for maximum flow rate and minimal damage to RBCs

Procedure

1. Identify Pt and obtain informed consent (consider cultural/religious beliefs).
2. Ascertain whether Pt has ever had a blood transfusion reaction.
3. Obtain venous access using an 18-gauge catheter and begin infusing 0.9% saline solution as prescribed by HCP. Use only 0.9% sodium chloride solution when administering blood products.
4. Maintain a separate IV line to administer medications and IV fluids.
5. Inspect blood bag for expiration date, damage, clots, leaks, discoloration, and bubbles.
6. Confirm ABO and Rh compatibility by comparing blood bank armband number with blood bag label and blood bank administration form; notify blood bank of any inconsistencies.
7. Have another nurse independently verify ABO and Rh compatibility (double-check).
8. Document beginning volume of each bag (volume varies).
9. Administer pre-transfusion medications, such as diphenhydramine, as ordered by HCP.
10. Begin transfusion within 30 min of receiving blood from blood bank.
11. Begin transfusion slowly and remain with Pt for the first 15 min to assess for transfusion reaction; if no evidence of reaction, transfuse at ordered rate.
12. Transfusions should not exceed 4 hr (septicemia risk); change tubing every 4–6 hr and after each unit of blood. Notify HCP if Pt has fever before transfusion.
13. Monitor VS, temperature, renal, circulatory, and respiratory status before transfusion, within 15 min of beginning transfusion, and every hour until 1 hr after completion.

Blood Products

Product	Components	Indications
Whole Blood	• Contains all blood products	• Rarely used • May be given emergently to a hemorrhaging Pt
Packed Red Blood Cells (PRBCs)	• No clotting factors or platelets, 80% plasma removed	• Acute and chronic anemia • Blood loss
Platelets	• Usually given in pools of 6–10 units	• Increase low platelet counts • Coagulopathies • One unit generally increases platelet count by 6000 units
Fresh Frozen Plasma (FFP)	• Plasma and clotting factors	• Replace clotting factors, e.g., after multiple transfusions (>6 units PRBCs) • Reverse effects of Coumadin (warfarin)
Cryoprecipitate	• Clotting factors	• Hemophilia, fibrinogen deficiency, DIC

With the exception of normal saline, do not add medications or IV fluids to blood products.

NCLEX Blood Specimen—Arterial Blood Gas

Supplies

- ABG collection kit
- Ice
- Pt label
- Rolled towel

Procedure

1. Allen Test: Ensure Pt has sufficient collateral circulation. Occlude blood flow, simultaneously, to radial and ulnar arteries. Instruct Pt to clench and release fist—hand should blanch. Release pressure over ulnar artery—return of color within 5 sec indicates sufficient collateral circulation.
2. Cleanse site over radial artery with alcohol swab.
3. Hyperextend Pt's wrist using rolled towel.
4. Palpate radial artery above insertion site.
5. Enter artery at a 45° angle, bevel up—ABG syringe should fill spontaneously (3–5 mL desired).
6. Remove needle, hold pressure for 5 min (10–15 min if Pt is anticoagulated), and apply pressure dressing.
7. Dispose of needle per standard precautions, expel air bubbles, and cap syringe. Gently roll syringe to mix specimen with heparin (do not shake).
8. Attach Pt label with nurse's initials, date, and time to specimen; place on ice, and transport to lab immediately.
9. Lab slip must include oxygen administration (room air if not on oxygen) and ventilator settings if applicable.

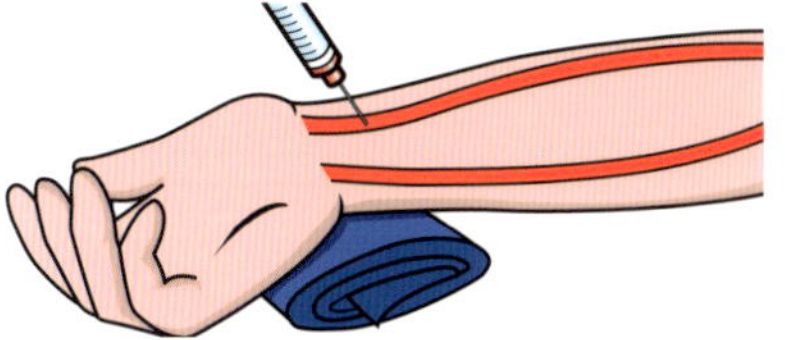

Blood Specimen—Finger Stick Blood Glucose (FSBG)

Supplies

- Glucometer
- Glucose monitor strip
- Warm compress
- Alcohol swab
- Lancets
- Cotton ball or gauze
- Small bandage
- Sharps container

Procedure

◎ Calibrate glucometer before obtaining specimen.

1. Follow manufacturer's guidelines for proper setup of glucometer before test; some glucometers require insertion of glucose strip in machine before application of blood to strip.
2. Select puncture site—preferred site is lateral aspect of fingertip. Avoid using the pad or distal tip or swollen, cold, or cyanotic sites. Avoid collecting specimen from same side as IV site. For infants, use lateral or medial side of either heel.
3. Promote capillary dilation as needed with warm compress for 5–10 min before puncture.
4. Cleanse site with alcohol swab and allow area to dry.
5. Position lancet perpendicular to dermal ridges and pierce skin—wipe away first drop of blood.
6. Apply second drop of blood to glucose monitor strip. Enhance blood flow by applying gentle, intermittent pressure, but avoid tight squeezing of finger.
7. Document results.
8. Apply gentle pressure to puncture site with cotton ball or gauze.

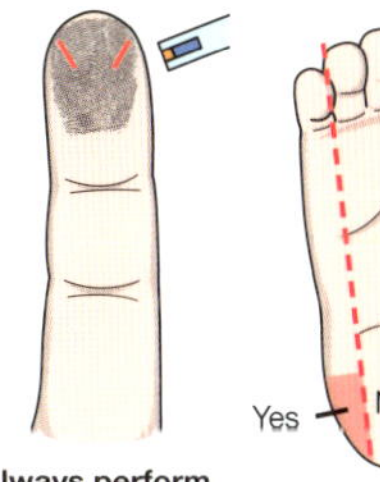

Finger Stick

Heel Stick

Blood Specimen—Venous Sample

Supplies

- Tourniquet
- Alcohol swab
- Appropriate-size catheter
- Gauze 2 × 2 or cotton ball
- Tape or Coban wrap
- Specimen tubes
- Pt label

Procedure

1. Select puncture site—antecubital (AC) fossa is most common site, but any vein below AC is acceptable. NCLEX Avoid previous puncture site areas for 24–48 hr; avoid collecting specimens above an IV site or sites that are infected or edematous. Avoid collecting from the same side as mastectomy, lymphadenectomy, dialysis shunts, or grafts.
2. Place tourniquet 3–4 in. above intended puncture site (preferably for no longer than 1 min).
3. Cleanse site with an alcohol swab from center out using a circular motion and allow to air-dry (use iodine if collecting blood alcohol level or blood culture specimens).
4. Insert needle, bevel up, at 15°–30°; stabilize needle and push specimen collection tube into needle holder; remove tourniquet when all specimens are collected.
5. Place gauze or cotton ball over puncture site, apply gentle pressure, remove needle, and secure dressing with tape.
6. Gently invert specimen tubes 3–5 times (do not shake).
7. Label specimen tubes with Pt's name, ID number, date, time, and your initials; send specimens to lab.

Order of Lab Draw

Color of Top	Additives	Uses
Yellow, yellow-black, green, or orange	SPS	Cultures on blood or body fluid
Red	No additive	As a discard tube when drawing blood using a butterfly needle (to remove air in tubing) or when drawing from an IV

Continued

Color of Top	Additives	Uses
Light blue	Sodium citrate	Coagulation tests
Red marble or gold	Gel separator and clot activator	Serum testing; most chemistry tests; immunology tests
Dark green	Sodium heparin	Blood chemistry such as whole blood and plasma testing
Light green	Lithium heparin and gel separator	Metabolic, lipid, and liver panels
Lavender	EDTA	Blood counts such as CBC, Hgb, Hct, glycosylated hemoglobin (A1C)
Light gray	Potassium oxalate and sodium fluoride	Glucose; glucose tolerance test, alcohol levels
Pale yellow	Acid citrate dextrose	Genetic testing; specialized testing

Tubes with additives must be thoroughly mixed.

Order of Draw concepts reprinted with permission from CLSI approved standard H3-A6, Procedures for the collection of diagnostic blood specimens by venipuncture, copyright 2007 (www.clsi.org)

Chest Tubes

Setup of Closed Chest Drainage System

Use strict aseptic technique during setup.

Water-Seal System

- **Two-chamber system:** Add NS or sterile water to second chamber (water-seal chamber) to level indicated.
- **Three-chamber system:** Add NS or sterile water to second chamber (water-seal chamber) to prescribed level.

Waterless System

- **Two-chamber system:** These systems are not used with suction, are ready to go, and require no additional setup.
- **Three-chamber system:** These systems are used with suction. Connect suction control chamber tubing to suction source.

Insertion

Pre-insertion

- Assist physician by positioning Pt, administering prescribed analgesics, and setting up and testing drainage system.

Post-insertion

- Position Pt to facilitate optimal drainage:
  - **Pneumothorax**: Semi-Fowler's or higher
  - **Hemothorax**: High-Fowler's
- Assess Pt for respiratory distress, assess insertion site for drainage and crepitus, and assess drainage system for complications.

Removal

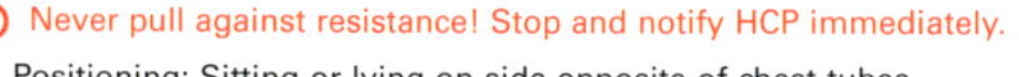

Never pull against resistance! Stop and notify HCP immediately.

1. Positioning: Sitting or lying on side opposite of chest tubes.
2. Administer prescribed analgesia 30 min before removal.
3. Remove sutures if used to secure chest tube in place.
4. Position and hold occlusive dressing at insertion site.
5. Instruct Pt to inhale deeply and hold breath.
6. Remove chest tube with one continuous, quick motion.
7. Secure occlusive dressing over insertion site.
8. Monitor Pt for signs of respiratory distress.

Troubleshooting

Supplies

- New drainage system
- Sterile connectors
- Toothless clamps
- Sterile occlusive dressing
- Tape
- Sterile water or saline
- Betadine swabs
- One-way (Heimlich) valve

NCLEX Air Leak

Intermittent bubbling during expiration is normal. Continuous bubbling in water seal chamber suggests an air leak.

1. Clamp chest tube using toothless clamps close to chest wall.
   - **If bubbling stops**: Air leak is within Pt or at insertion site. Unclamp chest tube, reinforce insertion site with occlusive dressing, and notify physician.

- **If bubbling continues:** Clamp chest tube (using second toothless clamp) at drainage unit.
  - If bubbling stops, air leak is in tubing. Replace tubing.
  - If bubbling continues, air leak is in drainage system. Replace system.

NCLEX Dislodgement From Patient

1. Immediately pinch skin opening together, then cover chest tube insertion site with sterile occlusive dressing. Tape three sides of dressing, leaving one side open for air to escape.
2. Notify physician, stat; continue to monitor Pt for distress.

NCLEX Disconnection in System

1. While preparing to reattach tube/connections: (1) submerge distal end of tube under 1–2 in. of sterile water or normal saline, or (2) attach a one-way (Heimlich) valve.
2. Clean exposed ends with Betadine swabs for 30 sec (air-dry for 30 sec). Reconnect and retape drainage system.
3. Replace all contaminated connections, including new drainage system, as quickly as possible to prevent a pneumothorax.

Cold Therapy

Avoid using cold therapy on extremities in Pts with peripheral neuropathy or diabetes.

- Review medical record for contraindications or conditions that may influence Pt's ability to tolerate cold applications.
- Establish baseline vital signs (including temperature) and assessment of area to be treated.
- Follow physician's orders regarding frequency and duration.
- Place absorbent pads underneath area to be treated.
- Apply cold therapy directly over injury.
- Assess skin condition every 5 min during therapy.
- Discontinue or adjust cold therapy if Pt complains of pain, burning sensation, or numbness.
- Discontinue cold therapy after 20 min of continuous application, or as ordered by physician.
- Provide instruction to Pt if cold therapy is to be managed by Pt.

Supplies

- Absorbent pads
- Cold therapy apparatus
- Plastic, ziplock bags
- Washcloth
- Pillowcase
- Ice and water

Ice Bag or Pack

1. Fill per manufacturer's guidelines (⅔ full if using plastic bag) and remove excess air before sealing.
2. If using chemically activated ice pack, activate by squeezing.
3. Wrap ice bag/ice pack in washcloth or pillowcase if it does not have a cloth-like exterior (e.g., if using plastic bag).

Electric Pump Cooling Device

1. Follow manufacturer's recommendations and fill reservoir with appropriate amounts of ice and water.
2. Wrap cooling pad in pillowcase if needed.
3. Apply cooling pad directly to (or around) body part.
4. Connect cooling pad hoses to cooling device.
5. Plug in and turn on cooling device, and adjust temperature according to physician's orders.
6. Position cooling device and secure hoses and electrical cord.

Dressing Change—Sterile

Supplies

- Sterile gloves
- Nonsterile gloves
- Irrigation solution
- Antiseptic solution
- Medicated ointment
- Prescribed dressing
- Sterile scissors
- Tape or Montgomery tie

Procedure

A. Remove old dressing using nonsterile gloves:
   1. Pull tape toward incision, parallel to skin.
   2. Be careful not to dislodge drainage tubes or sutures.
   3. Assess condition and appearance of wound including size, color, and presence of exudate, odor, ecchymosis, or induration. (See Wound Assessment.)
   4. Discard gloves and wash hands.

B. Using sterile technique, don face mask and sterile gloves, open supplies, set up a sterile field, and fill sterile containers with prescribed solutions.

C. Cleanse wound with prescribed solution:
   1. Start from area of least contamination—cleanse toward area of most contamination (use separate swabs).

2. Cleanse outward using circular motion around drains.
3. Apply antiseptic/medicated ointments as prescribed.

D. Apply prescribed dressing (see Dressing Types):
1. Cut dressings to fit around drain if present (use sterile scissors).
2. Reinforce with thick cover dressing (ABD or Surgipad).
3. Secure dressing with 2-in. tape, rolled gauze, or use Montgomery ties for frequent (every 4–6 hr) dressing changes.
4. Record date and time on paper tape and secure to dressing.

Dressings

Application Techniques

Dry: Apply dry, sterile gauze directly to wound and then cover with sterile 4 × 4 gauze or Surgipad.

Moist-to-dry: Soak sterile gauze in sterile solution and ring out excess. Apply moist gauze to wound, cover with dry, sterile 4 × 4 gauze, then cover everything with Surgipad or gauze.

Wound packing: Use sterile forceps and gently pack wound with moist, sterile gauze until all wound surfaces are in contact with moist gauze, including undermined areas. Do not allow moist gauze to touch surrounding skin, and do not pack wound beyond skin level. Cover with dry, sterile 4 × 4 gauze, then cover everything with Surgipad or gauze.

Dressing Types

Transparent: For superficial wounds, blisters, and skin tears. Ideal for stage I and II ulcers.

- Waterproof; maintains moisture and prevents bacterial contamination.

Hydrogel: For dry, sloughy wound beds; cleanses and debrides. Ideal for stage II, III, and IV ulcers.

- Provides moist wound environment. Reduces pain and soothes.

Hydrocolloid: For wounds with low-to-moderate exudate. Ideal for stage II and III ulcers.

- For autolytic debridement of dry, sloughy, or necrotic wounds.

Alginate: For wounds with moderate-to-heavy exudate. Ideal for stage III and IV ulcers.

- Available in pads, ropes, or ribbons.

Foam: Used after debridement or desloughing of ulcers. Ideal for stage III and IV ulcers. Highly absorbent. May be left on for 3–4 days.

- For wounds with heavy exudate, deep cavities, or weeping ulcers.

Insertion of NG Tube

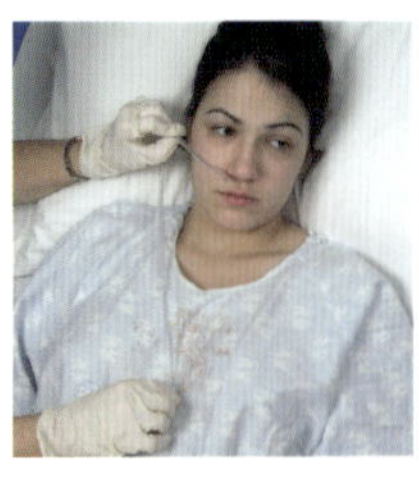

1. **Positioning**: Upright in high-Fowler's—maintain a chin-to-chest posture during insertion (reduces chance of intubating trachea).
2. Measure tube from tip of nose to earlobe, then down to xiphoid. Mark point on tube with tape.
3. Lubricate tube with water-soluble lubricant (petroleum-based jelly degrades PVC tubing).
4. Insert tube through nostril until you reach previously marked point on tube. Instruct Pt to take small sips of water during insertion to help pass tube.
5. Secure tube to Pt's nose with tape, being careful not to block nostril. Tape tube 12–18 in. below insertion line and then pin tape to Pt's gown. Allow slack for movement.
   NCLEX Double lumen (Salem sump): Secure (unclamped) above level of stomach.
6. Position HOB at 30°–45° to minimize risk of aspiration.
7. Document type and size of NG tube, which nostril, how Pt tolerated procedure, how tube placement was confirmed, and whether tubing was left clamped or attached to feeding pump or suction.

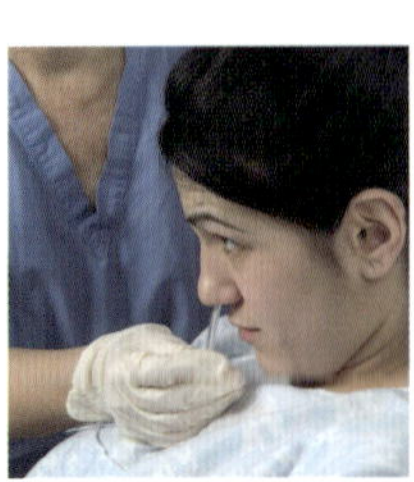

◎ Withdraw tube immediately if Pt becomes cyanotic or develops dyspnea. An inability to speak suggests intubation of trachea.

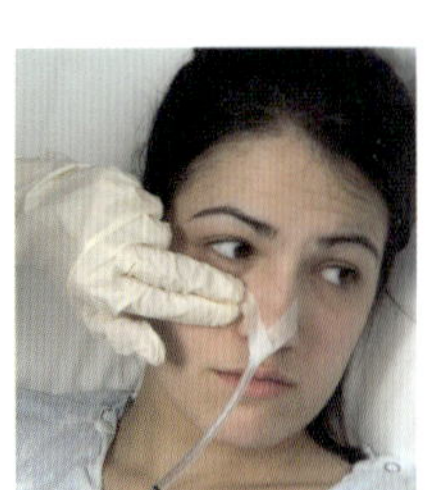

NCLEX Confirming Proper Placement of NG Tube

- Always use more than one method to ensure proper tube placement; never rely on just one method.
- For small-bore nasointestinal tubes (may collapse under pressure when aspirating), or if incorrect placement is otherwise suspected, confirm placement by x-ray.

Observation

- Verify marking on tube is at Pt's nostril.
- Compare length of exposed tube to initial length documented in Pt's chart.

Aspiration

- Aspirate gastric contents using a 20-mL syringe.
- Gastric aspirate should appear green with particulate matter or brown if blood is present.

Measurement of pH

- Dip litmus paper into gastric aspirate.
- A pH of 1–3 (<5) suggests placement in stomach.

Auscultation

- Method is controversial and is not used in some institutions.
- Inject 20 mL of air into tube while auscultating abdomen.
- A loud gurgle of air suggests placement in stomach.

Removal of NG Tube

- **Positioning:** Upright, 30°–45°
  1. Discontinue suction.
  2. Unpin tube from Pt's gown; remove tape from Pt's nose.
  3. Confirm placement; clear tube by flushing with 50 mL of air.
  4. Clamp tube (prevents aspiration), instruct Pt to hold breath, and remove tube in one gentle, but swift motion.
  5. Assess for signs of aspiration.

Oral Care—Unconscious or Debilitated Patient

◎ Ensure suction is set up and working.

◎ Avoid tap water in ventilated Pts—use saline.

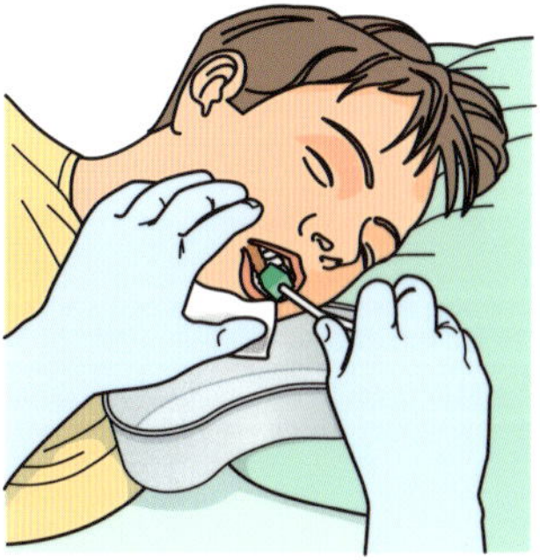

- **Positioning:** Side-lying—HOB down.
  1. Position absorbent pad beneath Pt's head.
  2. Position emesis basin under Pt's mouth.
  3. Use a bite block or padded tongue depressor to assist with holding Pt's mouth open.
  4. Apply toothpaste to moistened toothbrush.
  5. Brush teeth in the normal manner: (a) Hold bristles at a 45° angle to the gum line. Use short, circular motions and brush inner and outer tooth surfaces including gum line. (b) Brush biting surfaces back and forth. (c) Brush Pt's tongue.
  6. Draw up 10 mL water or approved mouthwash and gently rinse along sides of Pt's mouth—suction as needed or allow rinse to drain into basin.
  7. Clean soft tissues of the oral cavity per institutional policy—use a different swab for each area.
  8. Apply water-soluble lip moisturizer.
  9. Dry Pt's face and mouth, and reposition as needed.

Ostomy Care

Types of Ostomies

- **Colostomy**: May be permanent or temporary. Used when only part of large intestine is removed. Commonly placed in sigmoid colon, a stoma is made from large intestine and is larger in appearance than an ileostomy. Contents range from firm to fully formed.
- **Ileostomy**: May be permanent or temporary. Used when entire large intestine is removed. A stoma is made from small intestine and is smaller than a colostomy. Contents range from pastelike to watery.

Applying or Changing an Ostomy Bag

- **Positioning**: Supine.
  1. Don gloves and gently remove old pouch.
  2. Discard gloves, wash hands, and don new pair of gloves.
  3. Wash area around stoma with soapy water; dry skin completely.
  4. Inspect appearance of stoma and condition of skin, and note amount, color, and consistency of contents and presence of unusual odor. (Note: A healthy stoma should be pink-red, and peristomal skin should be free from any redness or ulceration.)
  5. Cover exposed stoma with gauze pad to absorb drainage.
  6. Apply skin prep in circular motion; allow 30 sec to air-dry.
  7. Apply skin barrier in circular motion.
  8. Measure stoma using stoma guide and cut ring to size.
  9. Remove paper backing from adhesive-backed ring, center ring over stoma, and gently press it to skin.
  10. Smooth any wrinkles to prevent seepage of effluent.
  11. Center faceplate of bag over stoma and gently press down until closed.
  12. Document appearance of stoma; condition of skin; amount, color, and consistency of contents; and presence of any unusual odor.

 Use supplemental oxygen judiciously in Pts with COPD.

<table>
<tr><th>Device</th><th>Rate (LPM)</th><th>FiO_2</th></tr>
<tr><td rowspan="6">Nasal Cannula
• For lower percentage supplemental oxygen.
• Flow rate of 1–6 L/min.
• Delivers 25%–45% oxygen.
• Pt can eat, drink, and talk.
• Extended use can be very drying; use humidifier.</td><td>1</td><td>25%</td></tr>
<tr><td>2</td><td>29%</td></tr>
<tr><td>3</td><td>33%</td></tr>
<tr><td>4</td><td>37%</td></tr>
<tr><td>5</td><td>41%</td></tr>
<tr><td>6</td><td>45%</td></tr>
<tr><td rowspan="5">Simple Face Mask
• For higher percentage supplemental oxygen.
• Flow rate of 6–10 L/min.
• Delivers 35%–60% oxygen.
• Lateral perforations permit exhaled CO_2 to escape.
• Permits humidification.</td><td>6</td><td>35%</td></tr>
<tr><td>7</td><td>41%</td></tr>
<tr><td>8</td><td>47%</td></tr>
<tr><td>9</td><td>53%</td></tr>
<tr><td>10</td><td>60%</td></tr>
<tr><td rowspan="2">Nonrebreather Mask
• For high-percentage FiO_2.
• Incorporates a reservoir bag.
• Flow rate of 10–15 L/min.
• Delivers up to 100% oxygen.
• One-way flaps prevent entrainment of room air during inspiration and retention of exhaled gases (namely, CO_2) during expiration.</td><td>10–15</td><td>80%–100%*</td></tr>
<tr><td colspan="2">* Removal of both flaps results in lower (80%–85%) FiO_2.
* Removal of one flap results in higher (85%–90%) FiO_2.
* Having both flaps in place results in maximum (95%–100%) FiO_2.</td></tr>
<tr><td rowspan="6">Venturi Mask (venti-mask)
• For precise titration of percentage of oxygen.
• Flow rate of 4–8 L/min.
• Delivers 24%–60% oxygen.
• Uses either a graduated dial or colored adapters selected to deliver desired FiO_2.</td><td>Blue</td><td>24%</td></tr>
<tr><td>White</td><td>28%</td></tr>
<tr><td>Orange</td><td>31%</td></tr>
<tr><td>Yellow</td><td>35%</td></tr>
<tr><td>Red</td><td>40%</td></tr>
<tr><td>Green</td><td>60%</td></tr>
</table>

Continued

Bag-Valve-Mask (BVM)

- For manual ventilation of Pt who has no or ineffective respirations.
- Can deliver 100% oxygen.
- Appropriate mask size and fit are essential to create good seal—hold mask with thumb and index finger; grasp underneath ridge of jaw with remaining three fingers.

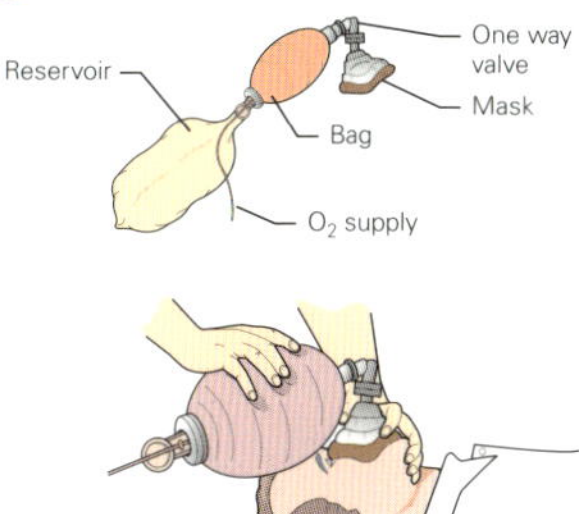

Humidified Systems

- For Pts requiring long-term oxygen therapy to prevent drying of mucous membranes.
- Setup may vary between brands; fill canister with sterile water to recommended level, attach to oxygen source, and attach mask or cannula to humidifier.

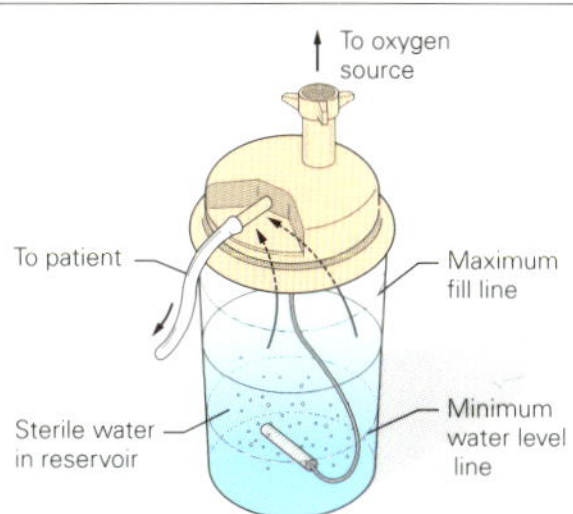

Transtracheal Oxygenation

- For Pts with a tracheostomy who require long-term oxygen therapy and/or intermittent, transtracheal aerosol treatment.
- Ensure proper placement (over stoma, tracheal tube).
- Assess for and clear secretions as needed.
- Assess skin for irritation.

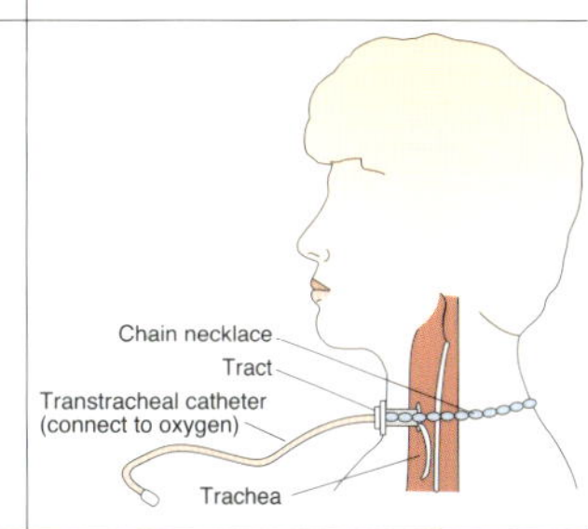

Pulse Oximetry

SpO_2	Intervention
>95%	• Considered normal and generally requires no invasive intervention.* • Continue routine monitoring of Pt.
91%–94% NCLEX	• Considered borderline.* • Assess and adjust probe placement. • Begin oxygen at 2 L/min titrated to SpO_2 >95%.
85%–90% NCLEX	• Elevate head and encourage Pt to cough and breathe deeply. • Assess airway and suction as needed. • Administer oxygen and titrate to SpO_2 >95%. • If condition fails to improve, assist ventilations manually and prepare to intubate.
<85%	• Administer 100% oxygen, set Pt upright, encourage coughing and deep breathing, and suction as needed. • Assist ventilations manually and prepare to intubate if condition fails to improve. • Consider reversal agents for possible drug-induced respiratory depression.

*Consider readings within overall context of Pt's medical history and physical exam. NEVER withhold treatment based solely on a "normal" SpO_2 reading.

Conditions That May Produce False Readings

False High Readings	False Low Readings
• Anemia • Alkalosis • CO poisoning • Hypovolemia • Pt movement	• Cool extremities • Drugs (vasoconstrictors) • Nail polish/nail infection • Pt movement • Poor peripheral circulation • Raynaud disease

NCLEX Restraints

Restraints are used only to protect Pt or staff from injury and should NEVER be used for convenience or punishment.

Types of Restraints

Safety-oriented restraints: Bed rails, wheelchair trays, mittens to prevent infants from scratching themselves.
Physical restraints: Fabric body holders, straightjackets, safety vests and jackets (e.g., Posey vest), limb restraints, and papoose boards for infants.
Chemical restraints: Medication administered to sedate or restrict the Pt's movements; use is highly restricted; most often used during surgical procedures.

Safety Guidelines

- Use the least invasive method needed to protect Pt or staff.
- Pt should be restrained in an anatomically correct position.
- All bony prominences should be adequately padded.
- Restraints should not interfere with circulation or treatment.
- Restraint should be secured to bed frame—never to hand rails.
- Secure all physical restraints using quick-release slipknots.
- Call light should be easily accessible to Pt.
- You should be able to fit two fingers easily under restraints.
- Assess restraint sites (e.g., skin, distal CSM) every 15 min.
- Physical restraints should be removed every 2 hr if possible—for aggressive Pts, remove only one restraint at a time.

NCLEX Alternatives to Restraints

- Provide regular orientation to reality and diversional activities.
- Encourage family to be involved with diversion and supervision.
- Move Pt closer to nurse's station.
- Use pressure-sensitive alarms in beds and chairs or sitters.
- Monitor Pt more frequently, and respond to call lights promptly.
- Conceal tubes and lines with pajamas or scrubs.
- Allow ample opportunity for supervised ambulation and toileting; avoid overstimulation.

Laws Pertaining to Restraints

- Alternative methods to promote safety should be attempted before using restraints; safety should be the nurse's priority.
- A physician's order must be obtained before restraining Pt and is valid for a maximum of 24 hr; in an emergency, an order must be obtained within 24 hr of restraint.
- Restraint orders must be reassessed by the ordering provider and reordered every 24 hr.
- Once a Pt is restrained, the nurse is responsible for the Pt's safety and well-being, and care should be appropriate for the type and severity of the restraint.
- Failure to properly monitor a restrained Pt may result in criminal and/or civil prosecution.
- Family should be notified to obtain consent if clinically reasonable.
- All interventions and Pt responses related to the use of restraints should be carefully documented.

Common Reasons for Using Restraints

- To prevent injury from falls.
- To prevent a confused Pt from roaming through the health-care facility endangering himself/herself.
- To prevent a confused Pt from trying to remove medically necessary tubes, IV lines, or protective dressings.
- To reduce risk for falls when a Pt has an unsteady gait.
- To prevent a Pt from inflicting self-harm or injury (suicidal).
- To prevent a Pt from inflicting harm upon health-care workers, other Pts, and/or visitors (homicidal).
- To ensure infant/child safety when a child cannot remain still during procedures; to prevent a child from hurting himself/herself.

SBAR—Communication Technique

Situation-Background-Assessment-Recommendation (SBAR) technique provides a framework for communication between members of the health-care team about a Pt's condition.

◎ Before calling physician, have available the Pt's chart, list of current medications, allergies, IV fluids, most recent vital signs, lab and other diagnostic tests with previous tests (if available) for comparison, and code status.

S	**Identify SITUATION you are calling about:** • Identify self, unit, Pt name, and room number. • Identify admitting physician if speaking to resident on call or physician. • Briefly state the presenting problem: What it is, time of onset, and severity.
B	**Describe BACKGROUND information related to situation:** • Admitting diagnosis, recent surgeries, code status. • Vital signs and pertinent assessment data. • Medications, allergies, IV fluids, lab and diagnostic test results.
A	**Describe ASSESSMENT of situation:** • What do you see? • What is your impression? • Examples may include allergic reaction, bleed, infection, MI, etc.
R	**Present RECOMMENDATION on what you would like:** • Pt needs to be seen now. • Order change or new orders. • Physician input.

Developed by Michael Leonard, MD, Doug Bonacum, and Suzanne Graham at Kaiser Permanente of Colorado, Evergreen, Colorado, USA

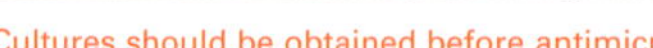

General Guidelines

NCLEX Cultures should be obtained before antimicrobial therapy.

Expectorated Specimens

1. **Positioning:** Upright position; provide over-bed table.
2. Instruct Pt to brush teeth or rinse mouth before specimen collection to avoid contamination with normal oral flora.
3. Instruct Pt to take 2–3 deep breaths and then cough deeply.
4. Sputum should be expectorated directly into a sterile container.
5. NCLEX Label specimen container and immediately send to lab.

Suctioned Specimens (Sputum Trap)

1. **Positioning**: Semi-Fowler's position if Pt is conscious, lateral position if unconscious.
2. If indicated, preoxygenate with 100% oxygen as ordered by health-care provider.
3. Open sterile suction package and set up sterile container; pour in sterile saline solution.
4. Attach sputum trap to suction source.
5. Turn on wall unit suction device to 100–200 mm Hg for adult client, 95–110 mm Hg for child, or 50–95 mm Hg for infant, or turn on portable unit to 10–15 mm Hg for adult, 5–10 mm Hg for child, or 2–5 mm Hg for infant.
6. Don sterile gloves; grasp sterile suction catheter with dominant (sterile) hand, and connect to sputum trap with nondominant hand (no longer sterile).
7. Moisten catheter by dipping into container of sterile saline; occlude suction control port to check suction.
8. Gently insert sterile suction catheter through nasopharynx, endotracheal tube, or tracheostomy; leave suction off by leaving suction control port open. Never apply suction as catheter is introduced.
9. Insert suction catheter just far enough to stimulate a cough reflex (shallow); apply suction by occluding suction control port with thumb; maintain sputum trap in an upright position during suctioning; suction for 5–10 sec, collecting 2–10 mL sputum.
10. Release suction (open suction control port) and remove catheter.
11. If sputum is thick and remains in suction catheter, suction a small amount of saline to flush specimen into sputum trap.

12. Disconnect sputum trap; if additional suction is needed, connect sterile suction catheter to suction tubing and suction as needed. (See Suctioning later in this section.)
13. Close sputum trap by looping rubber tubing over onto suction port on sputum trap.
14. NCLEX Attach Pt label with date, time, and your initials; send to lab immediately.

Throat Culture

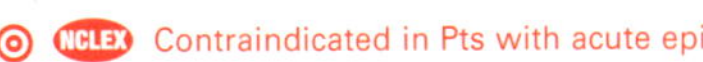

1. **Positioning:** Head tilted back with mouth open.
2. Use tongue depressor to prevent contact with tongue or uvula.
3. Using a sterile culturette, swab both tonsillar pillars and oropharynx.
4. Place culturette swab into culturette tube, and squeeze bottom to release liquid transport medium.
5. Ensure swab is immersed in liquid transport medium.
6. Label specimen container—send to lab at room temperature.

NCLEX Standard Precautions

Hand Hygiene

- Perform before and after every Pt contact.
- Wash hands with soap and warm water for 20 sec.
- Alcohol-based hand sanitizers are acceptable before and after casual Pt contact (e.g., obtaining vital signs).

Personal Protective Equipment (PPE)

- **Gloves:** Use whenever contact with body fluids, mucous membranes, nonintact skin, or contaminated items is likely. Remove and discard immediately after use—before touching noncontaminated items or caring for other Pts.
- **Eye protection and masks:** Use during Pt care activities likely to generate splashes or sprays of body fluids. Respirator (N95-type): Use as part of airborne precautions when caring for Pts infected or suspected to be infected with highly infectious pathogens transmitted by airborne particles (e.g., TB, measles).
- **Gown:** Use during Pt care activities to protect exposed skin and clothing when contact with body fluids is likely.

Removing Soiled Gloves

1. Without touching exposed skin, grasp palm of glove with other gloved hand and peel glove off, turning it inside out.
2. Hold removed glove in hand that is still gloved.
3. Without touching outside of remaining glove, slide 1–2 fingers inside cuff of remaining glove and peel second glove off, inside out, over first glove enclosing first glove completely.

Sharps—Linen—Refuse—Equipment

- Never recap used needles.
- Dispose of sharps in puncture-resistant containers.
- Place soiled linen and contaminated refuse in leak-proof bags—follow institutional policy regarding recycling.
- Disinfect and store reusable equipment after use.

Transmission-Based Precautions

- **Airborne**: Private, negative-airflow room, N95 mask, Pt to wear surgical mask on transport or if coughing excessively.
- **Droplet**: Private room, surgical mask, Pt to wear surgical mask on transport or if coughing excessively.
- **Contact**: Private room, gloves and gown during Pt contact.
- **Reverse isolation (to protect Pt)**: Private, positive pressure airflow room, surgical mask, restrict visitor access.

Stool—Specimen Collection

Preservatives are poisonous; avoid contact with skin.

Occult Blood (Hemoccult, Guaiac)

1. Open collection card.
2. Obtain small amount of stool with wooden collection stick and apply onto area labeled box A; the freshest sample possible will yield optimal results.
3. Use other end of wooden collection stick to obtain second sample from different area of stool and apply it onto area labeled box B; specimens should not come in contact with urine or toilet water.
4. Close card, turn over, and apply one drop of control solution to each box as indicated.

5. A color change is positive, indicating blood in stool.
6. Note: If Pt is collecting specimens at home, instruct Pt to collect specified number of specimens, keep them at room temperature, and drop them off in designated time frame.

Cysts and Spores—Ova and Parasites

1. Using attached spoon, place bloody or slimy/whitish (mucous) areas of stool into each container. Do not overfill containers.
2. Place specimen in empty container (clean vial) up to fill line; replace cap and tighten securely.
3. Place enough specimen in container with liquid preservative (fixative) until liquid reaches fill line; replace cap and tighten.
4. Shake container with preservative until specimen is mixed.
5. Write Pt ID information, date and time of collection on each container, keep at room temperature, and send specimens to lab immediately after collection.
6. If Pt is collecting specimens at home, instruct Pt to collect specified number of specimens, keep them at room temperature, and drop them off within designated time frame.

Suctioning

Closed System—Ventilated Patient

1. Place Pt on pulse oximeter during and after procedure.
2. Adjust the FiO_2 setting on the mechanical ventilator to 1.0.
3. ◎ Manual ventilation is no longer recommended, because it has been shown to be ineffective for providing delivered FiO_2 of 1.0.
4. Ensure that suction is turned on no higher than 150 mm Hg; suctioning pressure should be set as low as possible while effectively clearing secretions.
5. Stand with your nondominant hand toward Pt's head.
6. Insert suction catheter just far enough to stimulate a cough reflex (shallow).
7. Apply intermittent suction while withdrawing catheter and rotating 360° for no longer than 10–15 sec to prevent hypoxia.
8. Repeat until Pt's airway is clear.
9. Suction oropharynx after suctioning of airway is complete.
10. Hyperoxygenate Pt for at least 1 min especially in Pts who are hypoxemic; do not hyperventilate unless ordered.
11. Monitor Pt for adverse reactions/complications.
12. Rinse catheter in basin with sterile saline in between suction attempts (apply suction while holding tip in saline).
13. Rinse suction tubing when done, and discard soiled supplies.

1. Explain procedure and administer pain medication before suctioning.
2. Adjust bed to comfortable working position and lower closest side rail.
3. Place Pt in a semi-Fowler's position if conscious; lateral position if unconscious.
4. Place towel or waterproof pad across Pt's chest.
5. Turn on wall unit suction device to 100–200 mm Hg for adult client, 95–110 mm Hg for child, or 50–95 mm Hg for infant, or turn on portable unit to 10–15 mm Hg for adult, 5–10 mm Hg for child, or 2–5 mm Hg for infant.
6. Open sterile suction package and set up sterile container; pour in sterile saline solution.
7. Don sterile gloves; grasp catheter with dominant hand and connect to suction tubing with unsterile, nondominant hand.
8. Moisten catheter by dipping into container of sterile saline; occlude suction control port to check suction.
9. Estimate distance from earlobe to nostril and place thumb and forefinger of nondominant hand at that point on catheter.
10. Gently insert catheter alongside of mouth toward trachea to suction oropharynx or along floor of an unobstructed nostril toward trachea to suction nasopharynx; leave suction off by leaving suction control port open.
11. Never apply suction as catheter is introduced.
12. Apply suction by occluding suction control port with your thumb and gently rotate catheter as it is being withdrawn; do not suction for more than 10–15 sec at a time.
13. Flush catheter with saline and repeat suction as needed, waiting 20–30 sec between each attempt; alternate nares when repeated suctioning is required; never force catheter.
14. Encourage Pt to cough and breathe deeply between suctioning.
15. Remove gloves and dispose of gloves, catheter, and container.
16. Auscultate chest and listen to breathing to assess effectiveness of suctioning.
17. Document time of suctioning, look and amount of secretions, and character of Pt's respirations before and after suctioning.
18. Offer oral hygiene if needed.

Tracheostomy Care

- A tracheostomy is a surgically created opening in the trachea.
- A tracheostomy tube is placed in the incision to secure an airway and to prevent it from closing.
- Tracheostomy care is generally done every 8 hr and involves cleaning around the incision, as well as replacing the inner cannula of the tracheostomy tube.
- After the site heals, the entire tracheostomy tube is replaced once or twice a week, depending on the physician's order.

◎ Use sterile technique during procedure.

Supplies

- Tracheostomy kit
- Suction kit
- 0.9% saline solution
- Sterile gloves

Cleaning

1. Preoxygenate Pt with 100% oxygen and administer sedative if Pt is agitated; administer pain medication, especially during the first 4 days after surgery.
2. Remove gauze dressing from tracheostomy site and note the amount and color of drainage.
3. Perform tracheostomy and oro-nasopharyngeal suctioning.
4. Using sterile technique, clean skin around stoma and external portion of tube with hydrogen peroxide using cotton-tipped applicators. Note condition of skin and stoma.
5. If Pt has a disposable inner cannula, remove old cannula, discard, and insert new cannula.

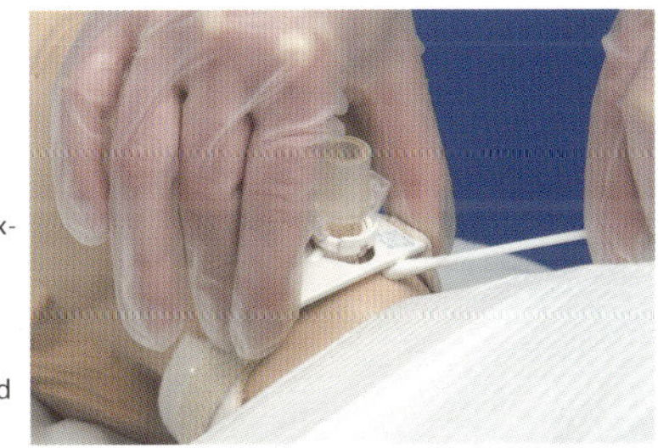

6. If Pt has a nondisposable inner cannula, remove inner cannula, clean with hydrogen peroxide, rinse with 0.9% saline solution, and reinsert; tap cannula against side of sterile container to remove excess solution; do not dry.
7. ◎ Only trained personnel should replace tracheostomy tube.
8. Suction Pt again if needed and assess respiratory status.

new tracheostomy dressing.
10. Replace Velcro straps (if soiled) as needed.

NCLEX Dislodgement

If Tracheostomy Is Less Than 4 Days Old

STAT intervention is required because tract can collapse suddenly—notify physician and RT STAT.

1. Open tracheostomy with a sterile hemostat, suction catheter, or sterile gloved finger to maintain airway and to keep edges of tracheostomy from collapsing.
2. If Pt cannot breathe, ventilate using BVM.
3. If you cannot be sure someone clinically prepared to reinsert tracheostomy tube will arrive within 1 min, call a Code.

If Tracheostomy Is More Than 4 Days Old

- Tract will be well formed and will not close quickly.
  1. Notify physician and RT that tube needs to be replaced.
  2. Obtain replacement tube if not already at Pt's bedside.
  3. Stay with Pt and prepare for insertion of new tube.

Tube Feedings

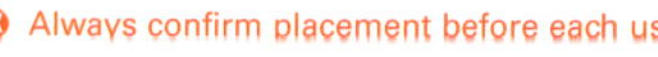

NCLEX Always confirm placement before each use.

- **Maintenance**: Flush with 30 mL water every 4–6 hr and before and after tube feedings, checking for residuals and administering medications.
- **Medication**: Dilute liquid medications with 20–30 mL water. Obtain all medications in liquid form. If liquid form is not available, check with pharmacy to see whether medication can be crushed. Administer each medication separately and flush with 5–10 mL water between each medication. Do not mix medications with feeding formula!
- **Residuals**: Check before bolus feeding, administration of medication, or every 4 hr for continuous feeding. Hold feeding if >100 mL and recheck in 1 hr. If residuals are still high after 1 hr, notify physician.

Administering Feedings

1. **Positioning**: HOB 30°–45° during and 30 min after feeding is complete to minimize risk of aspiration.
2. Follow manufacturer/institutional guidelines regarding type of feeding and operation of tube feeding delivery system.

3. NCLEX Confirm correct tube placement. (See Nasogastric Tube.)
4. Check residuals. (See Checking Residuals.)
5. Begin tube feeding at prescribed rate/interval as ordered.

Checking Residuals

◎ High residuals can indicate gastroparesis and intolerance to advancement to higher volume of formula.

◎ Check before each feeding, before administration of medication, or every 4 hr for continuous feeding.

1. Using 60-mL syringe, withdraw from gastric feeding tube any residual formula that may remain in stomach.
2. If residual volume is greater than predetermined amount (usually >100 mL), stomach is not emptying properly, and next feeding is withheld and rechecked in 1 hr.
3. If residuals are still high after 1 hr, notify physician.

NCLEX Tube Feeding—Complications

Complication	Common Causes and Interventions
Nausea, Vomiting, Bloating	• **Large residuals:** Withhold or decrease feedings. • **Medication:** Review meds and consult physician. • **Rapid infusion rate:** Decrease rate.
Diarrhea	• **Too-rapid administration:** Reduce rate. • **Refrigerated TF:** Administer at room temp. • **Tube migration into duodenum:** Retract tube to reposition in stomach and reconfirm placement.
Constipation	• **Decreased fluid intake:** Provide adequate hydration. • **Decreased dietary fiber:** Use formula with fiber.
Aspiration, Gastric reflux	• **Improper tube placement:** Verify placement. • **Delayed gastric emptying:** Check residuals. • **Positioning:** Keep HOB elevated 30°–45°.
Occluded tube	• **Inadequate flushing:** Flush more routinely. • **Use of crushed meds:** Switch to liquid meds.
Displaced tube	• **Improperly secured tube:** Retape tube. • **Confused Pt:** Follow institutional policy.

Condom Catheter Application

⊚ Use only materials supplied by manufacturer for securing catheter sheath to penis—failure to do so may result in compromised blood flow to the penis.

1. **Positioning**: Legs flat, slightly apart.
2. Establish baseline assessment of condition of penis.
3. Provide perineal care and dry thoroughly.
4. Refer to manufacturer's measuring guide to ensure correct sizing and application.
5. Ensure foreskin is not retracted in uncircumcised Pts.
6. Roll sheath onto penis, leaving 1–2 in. between tip of penis and end of condom catheter.
7. Secure sheath according to manufacturer's instructions.
8. Secure tubing to Pt's leg according to institution's policy.
9. Hang drainage bag on bed frame below level of the bladder.

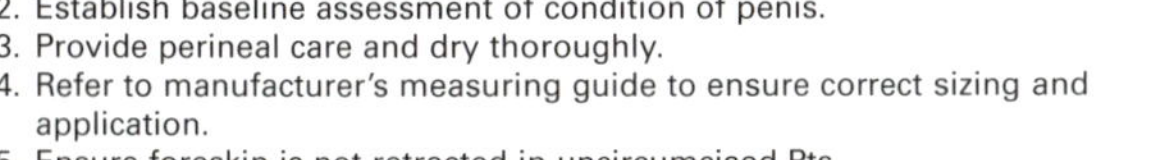

Indwelling and Straight Catheters

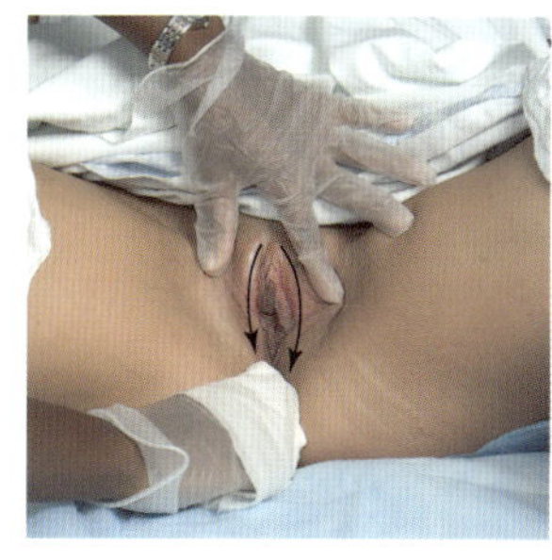

1. Positioning: **Female:** Knees up, legs apart; **Male:** Legs flat, slightly apart.
2. If placing indwelling catheter, check for leaks and proper inflation of balloon by filling with 5 mL sterile water. Remove water.
3. Lubricate catheter tip with water-soluble lubricant; saturate cotton balls with cleansing solution.
4. With nondominant hand (now contaminated) and using dominant (sterile) hand to hold swabs with sterile forceps:
   - Females: Hold labia apart; swab from front to back, in following order: (a) labia farthest from you, (b) labia nearest to you, and (c) center of meatus between labia. Use one swab per swipe.
   - Males: Retract foreskin; swab in a circular motion from meatus outward. Repeat 3 times, using a different swab each time.
5. Gently insert catheter (about 2–3 in. for female Pts and 6–9 in. for male Pts) until return of urine is noted. *Straight:* Collect specimen or drain bladder and remove and discard catheter. *Indwelling:* Insert an additional inch and inflate balloon.

   Uncircumcised males: Reposition foreskin after insertion.

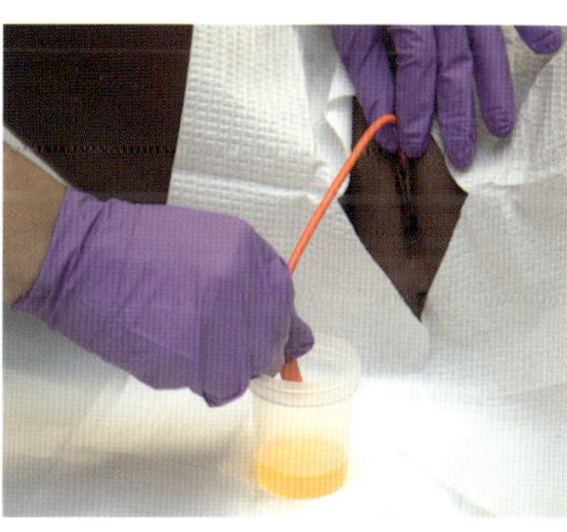

6. Attach catheter to drainage bag using sterile technique.
7. Secure tubing to Pt's leg according to institutional policy.
8. Hang drainage bag on bed frame below level of the bladder.

Urinary Catheter—Removal

1. Use a 10-mL syringe to withdraw all water from balloon. Some catheter balloons are overinflated or hold up to 30 mL; withdraw and discard water until no more water can be removed.
2. Hold a clean 4 × 4 at meatus with nondominant hand. With dominant hand, gently pull catheter. If you meet resistance, stop and reassess if balloon is completely deflated. If balloon appears to be deflated and catheter cannot be removed easily, notify physician.

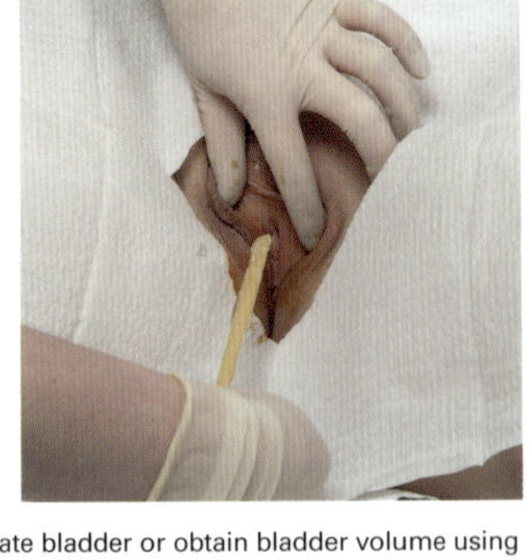

3. Wrap tip in clean 4 × 4 as it is withdrawn to prevent leakage of urine. Use a sterile 4 × 4 if a culture of catheter tip is desired.
4. Provide bedpan, urinal, or assistance to bathroom as needed.
5. Document time of removal and how Pt tolerated procedure.
6. Document amount and time of spontaneous void.
7. If Pt does not void within 8 hr, palpate bladder or obtain bladder volume using a bladder scanner and notify physician. Catheter may need to be reinserted.

Urine—Specimen Collection

Catheterized Patients

1. Ensure tubing is empty; clamp distal to collection port for 15 min.
2. Cleanse collection port with antiseptic swab; allow to air-dry.
3. Use a syringe to withdraw required amount of specimen.
4. Remember to unclamp tubing after specimen is collected.

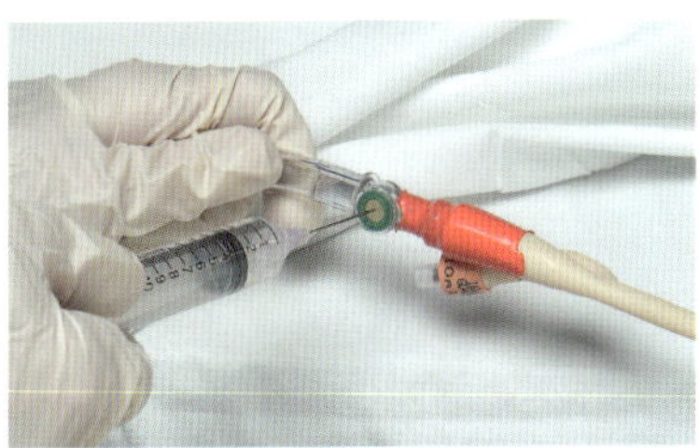

Clean-Catch (Midstream)

- Indicated for microbiological and cytological studies.
  1. Wash hands thoroughly.
     - **Male:** Cleanse meatus, pull back foreskin.
     - **Female:** Cleanse labia and meatus from front to back.
  2. Void small amount into toilet.
     - **Male:** Keep foreskin pulled back.
     - **Female:** Hold labia apart.
  3. Void into specimen collection container without interrupting flow of urine.
  4. Secure lid tightly.

First Morning

- Yields a very concentrated specimen for screening substances less detectable in a more dilute sample.
  1. Instruct Pt to void into specimen container upon awakening.

- Indicated for routine screening and may be collected at any time.
  1. Instruct Pt to void into specimen container.

Second Void

- Yields freshly produced urine to evaluate a Pt's current status (e.g., glucose and ketones).
  1. Instruct Pt to void, then have patient drink a glass of water.
  2. Wait 30 min; have patient void into a specimen collection container.

Timed (24-Hour Urine)

- Used to quantify substances in urine and to measure substances whose level of excretion varies over time.
- Ideally, collection should begin between 6:00 a.m. and 8:00 a.m.
- Keep specimen container refrigerated or on ice for entire collection period.
- Start time begins with collection and discard of first void.
  1. Instruct Pt to discard first void of day, and record date and time on collection container.
  2. Catheterized Pts: Time begins after bag and tubing have been replaced.
  3. Add each subsequent void to collection container.
  4. Instruct Pt to void at the same time the following morning and add it to collection container.
  5. Catheterized Pts: At 24 hours, empty remaining urine into collection container.
  6. This is the end of the 24-hour collection period.
  7. Record date and time, and send specimen to lab.

Ventilators—Patient in Distress

When ventilator alarms, always check Pt first!

- **Pt not in distress:** Check ventilator to determine source of problem.
- **Pt in distress:** Have RT/physician notified STAT and follow steps below—assist with reintubation as needed.

Ventilated Patient in Respiratory Distress

1. Disconnect ventilator tubing from ET tube and manually ventilate Pt.
2. Have RT/physician notified STAT if not already done.

Patient is Easy to Manually Ventilate

1. Ventilator is probable source of problem. Notify RT.
2. Manually ventilate Pt while RT assesses ventilator.

Patient is Difficult to Manually Ventilate

- **Dislodgement:** If tube dislodged, remove and manually ventilate Pt. Suction oropharynx to clear secretions.
- **Obstruction:** Suction ET tube to clear secretions. Notify RT. If unable to clear obstruction or pass suction catheter, extubate and manually ventilate (suction oropharynx as needed to clear secretions).
- **Pneumothorax:** If ineffective ventilation continues after airway, ET, and ventilator are all determined to be patent, inspect and auscultate Pt's chest. If there is unequal chest wall movement and/or decreased air movement on one side, it may be related to a tension pneumothorax (other causes may include an incorrectly positioned ET tube or atelectasis).
- **Equipment:** Inspect cuff for air leak (check cuff pressure if manometer available). Notify RT/physician if air leak cannot be fixed.

If ineffective ventilation continues and no physical or mechanical cause can be found, consider sedating Pt.

Alarm	Common Causes and Interventions
NCLEX Low-Pressure	**Causes:** System disconnects or leaks. 1. Reconnect Pt to ventilator. 2. Evaluate cuff and reinflate if needed (if ruptured, tube must be replaced). 3. Evaluate connections and tighten, or replace as needed. 4. Check ET tube placement (auscultate lung fields and assess for equal, bilateral breath sounds).
NCLEX High-Pressure	**Causes:** Resistance within the system such as a kink or water in the tubing, Pt biting ET tube, copious secretions, or plugged ET tube. 1. Suction Pt if secretions suspected. 2. Insert bite block as needed. 3. Reposition Pt's head and neck, or reposition tube. 4. Sedation may be required to prevent Pt from fighting vent, but only after you exclude physical or mechanical causes.
High Respiratory Rate	**Causes:** Anxiety or pain, secretions in ET tube or airway, or hypoxia. 1. Suction Pt. 2. Look for source of anxiety (i.e., pain, environmental stimuli, inability to communicate, restlessness). 3. Evaluate oxygenation.
Low Exhaled Volume	**Causes:** Tubing disconnect or inadequate seal. 1. Evaluate/reinflate cuff; if ruptured, ET tube must be replaced. 2. Evaluate connections; tighten or replace as needed; check ET tube placement, reconnect to ventilator.

Wound Culture

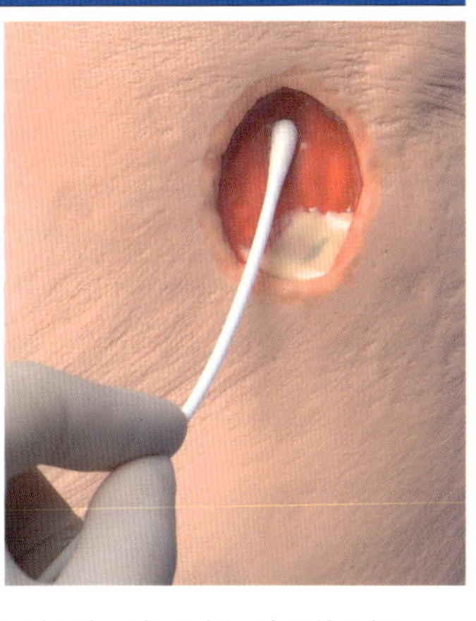

1. Remove old dressing if present.
2. Discard gloves, wash hands, and don new gloves.
3. Irrigate wound thoroughly with sterile saline or irrigation solution ordered by physician.
4. Discard gloves, wash hands, and don new gloves.
5. Swab healthy-looking area of wound bed:
   - **Levine technique**: Rotate sterile swab over a small (1-cm) area with sufficient pressure to express fluid from within the wound tissue.
   - **Zigzag technique**: While applying light pressure, swirl sterile swab between fingers, sliding swab from one edge of the wound to the other edge using 10-point zigzag pattern.
6. Place entire swab into culture tube (activate medium if needed) and secure lid tightly.
7. Transport specimen to lab per institutional policy.
8. Apply a new sterile dressing as ordered.

Normal Range Vital Signs

Age	RR	HR	SBP
Newborn	30–60	100–180	60–90
1–12 mo (infant)	30–60	100–160	87–105
1–2 yr (toddler)	20–40	80–110	85–102
3–5 yr (preschooler)	22–34	70–110	89–108
6–12 yr (school age)	18–30	65–110	94–120
13–17 yr (adolescent)	12–16	60–90	107–137
≥18 yr (adult)	12–20	60–100	90–>120

Temperature

Normal Core Temperature: 98.6°F–100.4°F (37°C–38°C)

Factors That Affect Vital Signs

Factor	HR	RR	SBP	Temp
Fever	↑	↑	Normal	↑
Anxiety	↑	↑	↑	Normal
Pain, Acute	↑	↑	↑	Normal
Pain, Chronic	↓	Normal	Normal	Normal
Acute MI	↓	↑	↓ (late)	Normal
Pulm. Embolus	↑	↑	↓	↑
Exercise	↑	↑	↑	↑
↓ H&H	↑	↑	↓	↓
↓ Blood Sugar	Normal/↑	Normal	Normal/↑	↓
↑ Blood Sugar	↑	↑/Deep	↓	↑
↑ WBC	↑	↑	↓ (sepsis)	↑
↑ K+	↓	Shallow	Normal/↑	Normal
↓ K+	↑	Shallow	↓	Normal
Narcotics	↓	↓	↓	↓
Beta Blockers	↓	↓	↓	Normal
Ca Channel Blockers	↓	↓	↓	Normal

Vital Sign Assessment

HR	1. Palpate pulse point for 30 sec and multiply by 2; count irregular pulse for full minute. 2. Compare right with left. 3. Document rate, rhythm, strength, and any right–left differences.
RR	1. **Position:** Comfortable; unaware respirations are being monitored. 2. Count respirations for 30 sec and multiply by 2; count irregular or labored respirations for full minute. 3. Document rate, depth, effort, rhythm, and any sounds; note whether heard on inspiration, expiration, or both.
BP	◎ NEVER use arm with dialysis shunt, injury, intra-arterial line, or same-side mastectomy or axillary surgery. AVOID arms with IV/VAD. 1. **Position:** Comfortable (sitting or HOB elevated) with arm slightly flexed and palm facing up, with forearm supported at heart level; ensure legs are not crossed. 2. Apply cuff snugly around upper arm, and ensure proper size and fit. 3. Place stethoscope over brachial artery and inflate cuff ~30 mm Hg over expected systolic pressure; slowly release cuff pressure. 4. Document point at which sound first heard (systolic) over point at which sound no longer heard (diastolic).
Temp	1. Follow manufacturer's recommendation for use of specific thermometer. Oral temp may be altered by recent hot or cold beverage, chewing gum, etc. 2. Document result and route.
Pain	1. Acute or chronic; etiology (disease or trauma). 2. Assess and document response to interventions. 3. Document score (0–10), location, OPQRST.

Health History	Biographic data, chief complaint, SAMPLE history, past medical history, family and social history, advance directives.
General Condition	Hygiene, state of well-being, nutrition, level of consciousness, emotional status, speech, affect, posture, gait, coordination, balance, gross deformities, mobility, range of motion, nonverbal cues.
Vital Signs	Temp, HR, RR, BP, and pain.
Skin	Temp, moisture, color, integrity, turgor, wounds, pressure ulcers, incisions, dressings, tubes and lines, lesions, scars, bruising, redness, body piercings, tattoos.
Head and Neck	**Head:** Shape and symmetry, condition of hair and scalp. **Eyes:** Conjunctiva, sclera, pupils, use of glasses or contacts. **Ears:** Pain, inflammation, drainage, hearing aids, hearing impairment. **Nose:** Drainage, congestion, sense of smell, NG tube, patency/equality of nostrils, nasal flaring, septal deviation. **Throat and Mouth:** Oral hygiene, odor, mucous membranes, gingival bleeding, lesions, condition of teeth, dentures, tongue, swallowing, tonsils. **Neck:** Stiffness, pain, range of motion, lymph nodes, thyroid, JVD, tracheal alignment, retractions.
Cardiovascular	Fatigue, exertional dyspnea, chest pain, dizziness, activity intolerance, edema, cyanosis or clubbing of nails, pulses, capillary refill, heart sounds, ECG tracing, presence of disease (CAD, CHF, MI, etc.).
Respiratory	Dyspnea, shortness of breath, cough, recent respiratory infections, lung sounds, oxygen therapy, oximetry, sputum characteristics, respiratory rate, rhythm, effort and pattern, disease (asthma, emphysema, etc.).
Gastrointestinal	Obesity, dietary habits, nausea, bowel patterns, stool characteristics, hemorrhoids, gastric tubes, ostomies, disease (reflux, celiac, IBS, etc.). Abdomen: Pain, distention, masses, herniations, scars, rigidity, bowel sounds.

Genitourinary	Hygiene, pain, sexual history, STDs, voiding pattern, nocturia, dysuria, discharge, lesions, urinary catheters. **Female:** Amenorrhea, vaginal bleeding, breast self-exams. **Male:** Erectile dysfunction, testicular pain, swelling, lumps, testicular self-exams.
Musculoskeletal	Pain, range of motion, muscle strength (p. 57), distal CSM, casts, amputations, prosthesis (stump condition), limb-length symmetry, deformities, physical limitations, assistive devices. **Extremities:** Pedal pulses, edema, ulcers, deep vein thrombosis (DVT).
Neurological	Pupils, mental status, cranial nerves, deep tendon reflexes, paralysis, paresthesia, stroke or seizure disorder, level of alertness and orientation, sleep pattern changes, clonus, Babinski sign in infants >18 mo.

Health History

Biographic Data	Record Pt's name, age, and date of birth, sex, race, ethnicity, nationality, religion, marital status, children, level of education, job, and advance directives.
Chief Complaint	What the Pt tells you (e.g., chest pain, nausea, abdominal pain). Use symptom analysis for chief complaint.
Past Medical History	Record childhood illnesses, surgical procedures, hospitalizations, serious injuries, medical problems, immunization, and recent travel or military service.
Medications	Prescription medications taken regularly as well as those taken only when needed (prn). Note: prn medications may not be used very often and are likely to be expired. Remind Pts to replace expired medications. Inquire about OTC drugs, vitamins, herbs, alternative regimens, and use of recreational drugs or alcohol.

Continued

	al changes, chemicals, latex, adhesives, etc. Determine type of allergic reaction (e.g., itching, hives, dyspnea).
Family History	Health status of blood relatives, as well as that of spouse/significant other. Obtain age and cause of death of deceased family members.
Social History	Assess health practices and beliefs, typical day, nutritional patterns, activity/exercise patterns, recreation, pets, hobbies, sleep/rest patterns, personal habits, occupational health patterns, socioeconomic status, roles/relationship, sexuality patterns, social support, and stress coping mechanisms.

Physical Assessment

- Always observe standard precautions.
- Before physical contact, perform a general survey.
- Evaluate all symptoms using the OPQRST approach.
- If Pt has an obvious problem, start at that point.
- Let Pt know your findings, and use this time to teach.
- Leave sensitive or painful areas until end of exam.

Different Approaches to Physical Assessment

- **Focused assessment:** Priority of assessment dictated by Pt's chief complaint (e.g., if Pt is complaining of CP, start with OPQRST).
- **Head-to-toe:** More complete, it assesses each body region (e.g., head and neck) before moving on to the next.
- **Systems assessment:** More focused, it assesses each body system (e.g., cardiovascular) before moving on to the next.

Focused Symptom Analysis (OPQRST)

Onset Origin	• When did symptom begin? • Was onset sudden or gradual? • Origin of symptom (e.g., injury, meal).
Provocation Precipitation Palliation	• Activity at or before onset of symptom. • Factors that worsen symptom. • Factors that alleviate symptom.
Quality	• Characteristics (dull, achy, sharp, etc.).
Radiation Region Related s/s	• Does symptom travel to another part of body? • Have Pt to point to source of symptom. • Document related symptoms (e.g., nausea, fever).
Severity	• If pain, rate on a scale of 0–10. • Is symptom mild, moderate, or severe?
Timing	• Ascertain duration of symptom. • Is symptom constant or intermittent?

Cardiovascular Assessment

History	CP, palpitations, syncope, fatigue, extremity changes (numbness, tingling, cold feet or hands, leg cramps, edema, lymphedema), activity intolerance, dyspnea on exertion, shortness of breath, orthopnea, number of pillows used for sleeping, hyperlipidemia, MI, CAD, PVD, DM, HTN, CHF, DVT, stents, CABG, pacemaker.
Medication	Beta/Ca-channel blockers, nitrates, diuretics, ACE inhibitors, anticoagulants, antiarrhythmics.
Neck	Venous distention (JVD), bruits, pulsations.
Chest	• Scars, symmetry, movement, deformity. • Auscultate lungs for pulmonary edema. • Compare apical and radial pulses for apical–radial pulse deficit (p. 5). • Heart valves for normal S_1, S_2 (lub, dub) heart sounds—abnormal sounds include extra beats (S_3, S_4), bruits, murmurs, pericarditic rubs, and artificial valve clicks. • PMI for pulsations, thrills, or heaves.
Abdomen	• Scars, edema, ascites, pulsations, and thrills.

- Nail beds for cyanosis and clubbing.
- Lower extremities for swelling and edema.
- Compare pulses right to left.
- Grade radial and pedal pulses.
- Grade peripheral edema.

Capillary Refill

Normal..<3 sec
Delayed..>3 sec

Pulse Strength Grading Scale

0...Absent
1...Weak
2...Normal
3...Full
4...Bounding

Cardiac Auscultation Sites

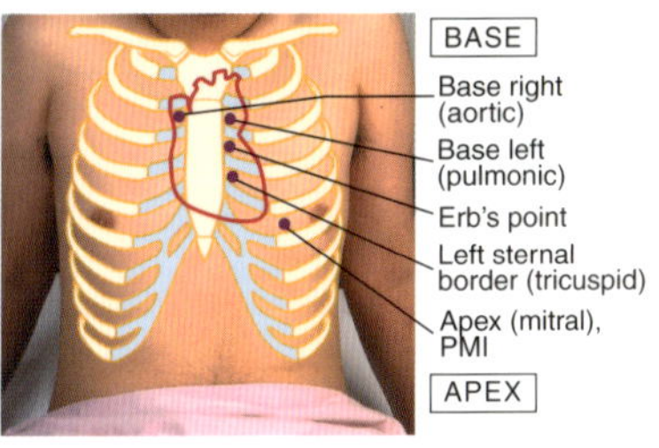

Deep Venous Thrombosis (DVT)

Never massage affected extremities.

- **History**: Recent surgery or fracture of leg or pelvis, prolonged bed rest, birth control pills, estrogens, smoking, recent childbirth.
- **Signs/symptoms**: Pain, tenderness, edema, swelling, redness, warmth.
- **Homans' sign**: Calf pain on dorsiflexion of foot.

Edema Grading Scale

Gently compress Pt's soft tissue with your thumb over a bony area for at least 5 sec; observe for indentation. If no indentation is noted, the Pt does not have pitting edema.

+1	**<2 mm** depression; disappears rapidly.
+2	**2–4 mm** depression; disappears in 10–15 sec.
+3	**4–6 mm** depression that lasts >1 min; swollen appearance.
+4	**6–8 mm** depression that lasts 2–5 min; grossly edematous.

NCLEX Gastrointestinal Assessment

History	Pain, bloating, changes in bowel pattern, diarrhea, constipation, changes in weight or appetite, indigestion, reflux, nausea, vomiting, stomach ulcers, *Helicobacter pylori*, hemorrhoids, GI bleed, UC, IBS, blood or mucus in stool, NSAID use.
Medication	Antacids, proton pump inhibitors, H2 antagonists, laxatives, antiemetics, antibiotics, antispasmodics.
Abdominal Pain (differential diagnosis)	• **RUQ**: Cholecystitis, hepatitis, MI, pancreatitis, perforated ulcer. • **LUQ**: Gastritis, peptic ulcer, MI, pancreatitis, splenic enlargement. • **RLQ**: Appendicitis, ectopic pregnancy, gynecological disease, renal calculi, testicular torsion, aortic dissection. • **LLQ**: Diverticulitis, colitis, aortic dissection, renal calculi, ectopic pregnancy, gynecological disease, testicular torsion. • **Epigastric**: MI, ulcer, pancreatitis. • **Diffuse**: Gastroenteritis, IBS, ischemic bowel, diabetic ketoacidosis.
Inspect (abdomen)	• Skin, distention, scars, obesity, herniations, bruising, pulsations.
Auscultate (bowel tones; before palpate)	• **Hypoactive**: Every minute. • **Normal**: Every 15–20 sec. • **Hyperactive**: As often as every 3 sec.

	• **Tympany:** Hollow organs (bowels). • **Resonance:** Air-filled organs (lungs). • **Flatness:** Dense tissue (muscle, bone).
Palpate (abdomen; after auscultate)	• Pulsations (aortic aneurysm). • Masses (stool, tumors). • Tenderness (appendicitis). • Rigidity (GI bleeding, guarding).

Abdominal Organs and Quadrants

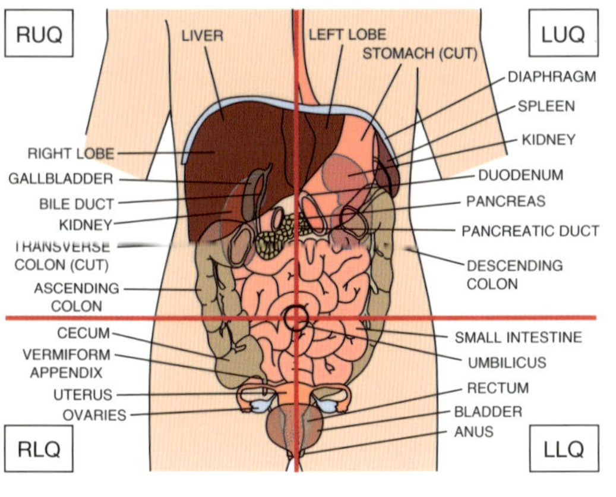

Genitourinary Assessment

History	• Kidney stones, blood in urine, dysuria, voiding pattern changes, itching, cancer (e.g., prostate, cervix, ovarian), UTI. • **Sexual history**: Sexual activity, use of protection against infection, method of birth control, multiple or same-sex partners, history of STD, ED (male Pts).
Medication	• Antibiotics, antifungals, antispasmodics, phosphodiesterase inhibitors (Viagra, Cialis, Levitra), analgesics.
Pain	• History of painful or burning urination? • **Female**: Dysmenorrhea (abnormally severe cramping during menstruation). • **Male**: Penis, testes, scrotum, and groin.
Lesions	• Blisters, ulcers, sores, warts, or rashes.
Breasts	• Symmetry, dimpling or edema, nipples (color, discharge, or inversion). • Lumps or tenderness (palpate in a concentric circle, outward from nipple, including axillae), presence of implants. • Breast self-exams?
Testicles	• Lumps, masses, or swelling (palpate scrotum and groin area). • Testicular self-exams?
Discharge	• **Female**: Assess for vaginal discharge and note color, odor, amount, and any associated symptoms. • **Male**: Inspect meatus for discharge and note color, amount, and any associated symptoms.
Menstruation	• Describe last period including date. • Do periods occur regularly? • Investigate bleeding other than normal period (frequency, quantity, symptoms).

Integumentary Assessment

History	Pruritus, rashes, changes in mole or lesion, nonhealing sores, changes in skin, hair or nails, eczema, psoriasis, acne.
Medication	• Topical creams, gels, or ointments such as antibiotic, antifungal, anti-inflammatory. • Oral medications such as antibiotics, antifungal and antiviral agents, biologics, immunosuppressants, and corticosteroids.

Appearance	• **Color:** Erythema, pallor, jaundice. • Bruising, scars, tattoos. • **Cyanosis:** Differentiation between central (lips, conjunctiva) and peripheral (nail beds, extremities) cyanosis. • Oral mucosa used for assessing color changes in dark skinned Pts. • Sclera used for assessing jaundice in Pts of Asian descent.
Hair and Scalp	• Texture and distribution. • Condition of scalp.
Nails	• Cyanosis, fungal infections. • Angle of attachment (normal, 160°; abnormal, >180°, indicating chronic pulmonary disease).
Temperature	• Coolness. • Warmth.
Moisture	• Diaphoresis. • Excessive dryness.
Turgor	• Time it takes skin to flatten after pinching. • Poor skin turgor is a sign of dehydration. • Sternum or forehead skin used in older Pts.
Lesions	• Presence and type of lesions or rashes. • Determining whether rashes blanch.
Wounds	• Pressure ulcers, surgical wounds. • Inspection of legs and feet of diabetic Pts.

Musculoskeletal Assessment

History	Pain (chronic or acute), stiffness, weakness, trauma, fractures, dislocations, deformities, limitations, immunizations (e.g., tetanus, polio).
Medications	Pain medications including prescribed narcotics, anti-inflammatory drugs, and OTC medications.
Mobility	• Gait, balance, coordination, limitations.
Spine	• Posture, spinal curvature. • Spinal deformities (scoliosis, kyphosis, lordosis).

Continued

Extremities	• Limb length discrepancy. • Grip strength. • Push-pull strength of feet. **Muscle Strength Grading Scale** **0**..............No muscle movement **1**..............Visible muscle movement, but no joint movement **2**..............Joint movement, but not against gravity **3**..............Movement against gravity, but not against resistance **4**..............Movement against resistance, but less than normal **5**..............Normal strength
Range of Motion	• Limitations and pain during movement of neck, shoulders, elbows, wrists, spine, hips, knees, and ankles. • Tests include: Flexion, extension, rotation, lateral bend, abduction, adduction, circumduction, supination, pronation, inversion, and eversion as applicable.

Neurological Assessment

Mental Status	• Affect, mood, appearance, behavior, and grooming. • Clarity of speech and coherence. • Alertness, lethargy, confusion, obtundation, stupor. • Orientation to person, place, time.
Motor	• Involuntary movements, muscle symmetry, atrophy. • Muscle Tone. • Flex and extend wrists, elbows, ankles, and knees; slight, continuous resistance to passive movement is normal. • Note any decreased (flaccid) or increased (rigid or spastic) muscle tone. • Motor strength. • Have Pt move against resistance. (See Muscle Strength Grading Scale in Musculoskeletal Assessment section.)

Continued

Reflexes	**Babinski's (Plantar) Reflex** • Stroke lateral aspect of sole of each foot with reflex hammer. • Normal response is flexion (withdrawal) of toes. • Positive (abnormal) Babinski's reflex is characterized by extension of big toe with fanning of other toes. **Clonus** • With knee supported in partially flexed position, quickly dorsiflex foot. • Rhythmic oscillations are positive for clonus. **Deep Tendon Reflexes** **0**........Absent **1+**........Diminished **2+**........Normal **3+**........Hyperactive without clonus **4+**........Hyperactive with clonus
Gait/Balance	Do not force Pts to attempt tasks beyond their limitations. • Observe gait while Pt walks across room and back. • Have Pt walk heel-to-toe or on heels in a straight line. • Have Pt hop in place on each foot. • Have Pt do shallow knee bend.
Coordination	Do not force Pts to attempt tasks beyond their limitations. **Rapid Alternating Movements** • Instruct Pt to tap tip of thumb with tip of index finger as fast as possible. **Point-to-Point Movements** • Instruct Pt to touch his or her nose and your finger alternately. Continually change position of your finger during test. **Romberg's Test** Be prepared to catch Pt! • Request that Pt stand with feet together, eyes closed for 10 sec. If Pt becomes unstable, test result is positive, indicating proprioceptive or vestibular problem. **Proprioception** • Instruct standing Pt to close eyes and alternate touching index fingers to nose.
Sensory	• Using your finger and a toothpick, instruct Pt to distinguish between sharp and dull sensations. • Compare left with right (Pt's eyes closed).

Cranial Nerves: Assessment

Nerve		Name	Function	Test
I	S	Olfactory	Smell	Have Pt identify familiar odors (e.g., coffee).
II	S	Optic	Visual acuity	Visual acuity (eye chart).
			Visual field	Peripheral vision.
III	M	Oculomotor	Pupillary reaction	Assess pupils for equality and reactivity to light.
IV	M	Trochlear	Eye movement	Have Pt follow your finger without moving head.
V	B	Trigeminal	Facial sensation	Touch face and assess for sharp and dull sensation.
			Mastication	Have Pt hold mouth open.
VI	M	Abducens	Abduction of eye	Have Pt follow your finger without moving head.
VII	B	Facial	Facial expression	Have Pt smile, wrinkle face, puff cheeks.
			Sense of taste	Differentiate between sweet and salty taste.
VIII	S	Acoustic	Hearing	Snap fingers close to Pt's ears.
			Balance	Feet together, arms at side with eyes closed for 5 sec.
IX	B	Glossopharyngeal	Swallowing and voice	Have Pt swallow and then say "Ah."
X	B	Vagus	Gag reflex	Use tongue depressor or swab to elicit gag reflex.
XI	M	Spinal accessory	Neck motion	Have Pt shrug shoulders or turn head against resistance.
XII	M	Hypoglossal	Tongue movement	Have Pt stick out tongue and move it from side-to-side.

B = both sensory and motor; M = motor only; S = sensory only.

Dermatomes

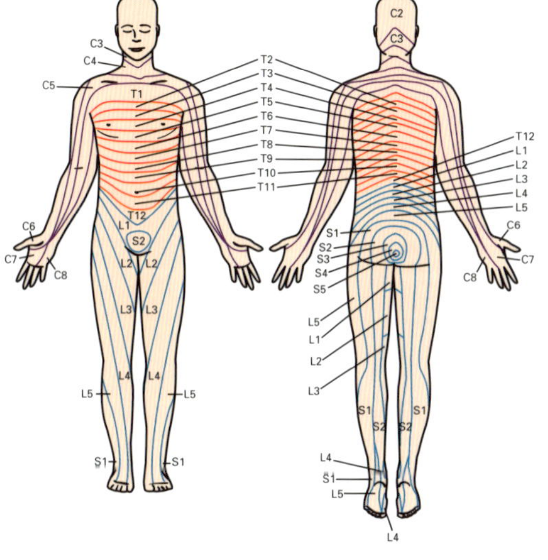

Determining Responsiveness: AVPU Scale

Alert	Pt is **A**lert and requires no stimulation.
Verbal	Pt responds only to **V**erbal stimulation.
Painful	Pt responds only to **P**ainful stimulation.
Unresponsive	Pt is **U**nresponsive to any stimulation.

Glasgow Coma Scale

	Adult–Child	Infant	
Eyes Open	Spontaneous	Spontaneous	4
	On command	**To voice**	3
	To pain	To pain	2
	Unresponsive	Unresponsive	1
Best Verbal	Oriented	**Coos, babbles**	5
	Confused	**Irritable, fussy**	4
	Inappropriate	**Cries to pain**	3
	Incomprehensible	**Grunts, moans**	2
	Unresponsive	Unresponsive	1
Best Motor	Obeys commands	**Purposeful**	6
	Localizes pain	Localizes pain	5
	Withdraws from pain	Withdraws from pain	4
	Abnormal flexion	Abnormal flexion	3
	Abnormal extension	Abnormal extension	2
	Unresponsive	Unresponsive	1

Reporting: The total GCS score should be broken down into its relative components (e.g., a GCS of 11 can be stated as E3V3M5).

Score: 13–14 indicates mild brain injury; 9–12 indicates moderate brain injury; and 3–8 indicates severe brain injury.

Teasdale, G., & Jeanett, B. (1974). Assessment of coma and impaired conciousness: a practical scale. *The Lancet, 304*(7872), 81–84. With permission.

Pupil Scale (mm)

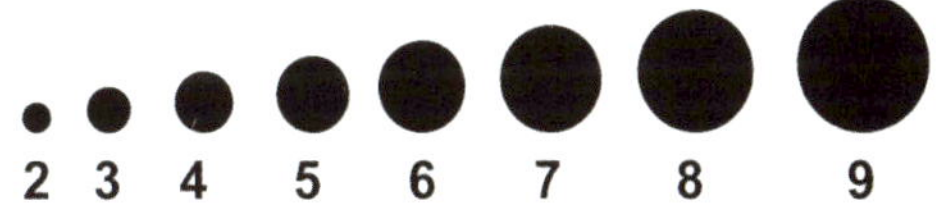

Nutritional Assessment

	Normal Findings	Suggests Malnutrition
Demeanor	Alert and responsive with positive outlook.	Lethargic, negative attitude.
Weight	Reasonable for build.	Underweight, overweight.
Hair	Glossy, full, firmly rooted, and uniform in color.	Dull, sparse, easily and painlessly plucked.
Eyes	Bright, clear, and shiny.	Pale conjunctiva, redness, dryness.
Lips	Smooth.	Chapped, red, and swollen.
Tongue	Deep red and slightly rough with one longitudinal furrow.	Bright red or purple, swollen or shrunken, with several longitudinal furrows.
Teeth	Bright and painless.	Cavities, painful, mottled, or missing.
Gums	Pink and firm.	Spongy, bleeding, receding.
Skin	Clear, smooth, firm, and not excessively dry.	Rashes, swelling, spots, excessive dryness, poorly healing wounds.
Nails	Pink and firm.	Spoon shaped, ridged, spongy bases.
Mobility	Erect posture, good muscle tone, walks without difficulty.	Muscle wasting, skeletal deformities, loss of balance.

Dehydration

	Mild	Moderate	Severe
Mentation	Alert	Lethargic	Obtunded
Capillary refill	2 sec	2–4 sec	>4 sec
Mucous membranes	Normal	Dry	Parched, cracks
Heart rate	Slightly ↑	Increased	Very increased
Pulse (character)	Normal, full	Thready	Faint, impalpable
Respiratory rate	Normal	Increased	Fast, hyperpnea
Blood pressure	Normal	Orthostatic	Decreased
Skin turgor	Normal	Slow	Tenting
Urine output	Decreased	Oliguria	Oliguria, anuria

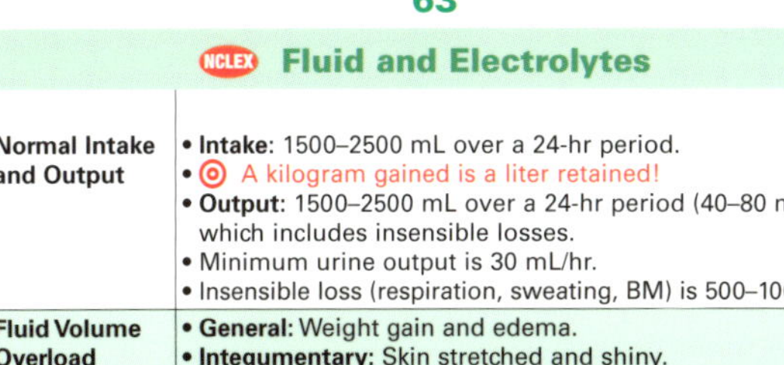

NCLEX Fluid and Electrolytes

Normal Intake and Output	• **Intake**: 1500–2500 mL over a 24-hr period. • A kilogram gained is a liter retained! • **Output**: 1500–2500 mL over a 24-hr period (40–80 mL/hr), which includes insensible losses. • Minimum urine output is 30 mL/hr. • Insensible loss (respiration, sweating, BM) is 500–1000 mL/d.
Fluid Volume Overload	• **General:** Weight gain and edema. • **Integumentary:** Skin stretched and shiny. • **CV:** Decreased hematocrit, widened pulse pressure, emptying of hand veins >5 sec, pulmonary edema, congestive heart failure. • **Urinary:** Polyuria, dilute urine (decreased output in renal failure). • **GI:** Nausea and anorexia (edema of bowel). • **CNS:** Deteriorating confusion.
Fluid Volume Deficit	• **General:** Weight loss. • **Integumentary:** Poor skin turgor, dry mucous membranes. • **CV:** Increased hematocrit, narrowing pulse pressure, filling of hand veins >5 sec, postural hypotension, tachycardia on standing. • **Urinary:** Oliguria, concentrated urine. • **GI:** Thirst, anorexia (decreased blood flow to intestine), longitudinal furrows on tongue. • **CNS:** Confusion and disorientation.

NCLEX Electrolyte Imbalance

Imbalance	Signs and Symptoms	Common Causes
Hypercalcemia Serum calcium level >10.5 mg/dL	Weakness, fatigue, anorexia, nausea, vomiting, constipation, polyuria, tingling lips, muscle cramps, confusion, hypoactive bowel tones.	Hyperparathyroidism or malignancies, thiazide diuretics, lithium, renal failure, immobilization, metabolic acidosis.

Continued

Imbalance	Signs and Symptoms	Common Causes
Hypocalcemia Serum calcium level <8.5 mg/dL	Anxiety, irritability, twitching around mouth, convulsions, tingling/numbness of fingers, diarrhea, abdominal/muscle cramps, arrhythmias.	Inadequate vitamin D intake, low albumin, renal failure, lactose intolerance, Crohn's disease, hyperthyroid, ↑ magnesium, acute pancreatitis.
Hyperkalemia Serum potassium level >5.0 mEq/L	Weakness, nausea, diarrhea, hyperactive GI, muscle weakness and paralysis, arrhythmias, dizziness, postural hypotension, oliguria.	Potassium-sparing diuretics, NSAIDs, renal failure, multiple transfusions, ↓ renal steroids, OD of potassium supplements.
Hypokalemia Serum potassium level <3.5 mEq/L	Anorexia, nausea, vomiting, fatigue, ↓ LOC, leg cramps, muscle weakness, anxiety, irritability, arrhythmias, postural hypotension, coma.	Anorexia, fad diets, prolonged NPO status, alkalosis, transfusion of frozen RBCs, prolonged NGT suctioning.
Hypermagnesemia Serum magnesium level >2.7 mg/dL	Muscle weakness and fatigue are most common, nausea, vomiting, flushed skin, diaphoresis, thirst, arrhythmias, palpitations, dizziness.	↑ Magnesium intake, chronic renal disease, pregnant women on parenteral magnesium for pre-eclampsia, Addison's disease.
Hypomagnesemia Serum magnesium level <1.7 mg/dL	Diarrhea, anorexia, arrhythmias, lethargy, muscle weakness, tremors, nausea, dizziness, seizures, irritability, confusion, psychosis, ↓ BP, ↑ HR.	Prolonged NGT suctioning, diarrhea, laxative abuse, malnutrition, alcoholism, prolonged diuretic use, DKA, digoxin.
Hypernatremia Serum sodium level >145 mEq/L	Confusion, fever, tachycardia, low BP, postural hypotension, dehydration, poor skin turgor, dry mucous membranes, flushed.	Fever, vomiting, diarrhea, ventilated Pts, severe burns, profuse sweating, diabetes insipidus, diuresis.
Hyponatremia Serum sodium level <135 mEq/L	Nausea, vomiting, abdominal cramps, diarrhea, headache, dizziness, confusion, flat affect, ↓ DBP, ↑ HR, postural hypotension, ↓ deep tendon reflex.	Diuretic use, vomiting, diarrhea, burns, hemorrhage, fever, diaphoresis, CHF, renal failure, hyperglycemia, ↑ ADH.

Pain Assessment

Characteristics of Acute and Chronic Pain

	Acute Pain	Chronic Pain
Onset	Current.	Continuous or intermittent.
Duration	<6 mo.	>6 mo.
ANS response	↑ HR, RR, BP, muscle tension, diaphoresis, pupillary dilation.	Rarely present.
Relevance to healing	Diminishes as healing occurs.	Continues long after healing.
Analgesics	Responsive.	Rarely responsive.

Focused Assessment—OPQRST

See Focused Symptom Analysis (OPQRST) on p. 51.

Pain Scales—FACES Pain Rating Scale*

0
NO HURT
2
HURTS LITTLE BIT
4
HURTS LITTLE MORE
6
HURTS EVEN MORE
8
HURTS WHOLE LOT
10
HURTS WORST

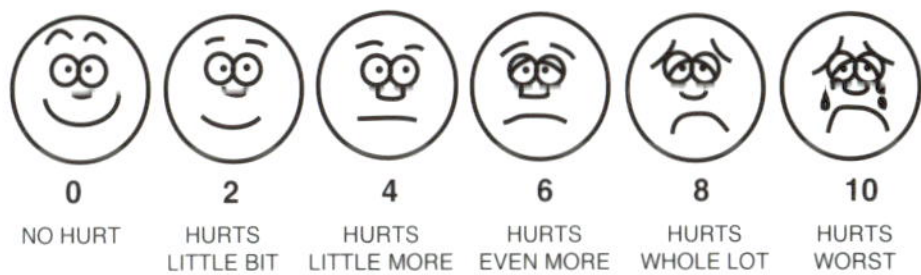

*For pediatric and non–English-speaking Pts.

Source: From Hockenberry, M. J., & Wilson, D. (2009). *Wong's essentials of pediatric nursing* (8th ed.). St. Louis, MO: Mosby. Used with permission. Copyright Mosby.

Spanish Numerical Pain Scale

0	2	4	6	8	10
Cero	*Dos*	*Quatro*	*Seis*	*Ocho*	*Diez*

← *Ningún dolor* (no pain) (much pain) *Mucho dolor* →

Pain Scales—FLACC Pain Scale for Pediatric Patients

Face	
• No particular expression or smile.	**0**
• Occasional grimace or frown; withdrawn; uninterested.	**1**
• Frequent to constant quivering chin, clenched jaw.	**2**
Legs	
• Normal position or relaxed.	**0**
• Uneasy, restless, tense.	**1**
• Kicking, or legs drawn up.	**2**
Activity	
• Lying quietly, normal position, moves easily.	**0**
• Squirming, shifting back and forth, tense.	**1**
• Arched, rigid or jerking.	**2**
Cry	
• No cry (awake or asleep).	**0**
• Moans with whimpers; occasional complaint.	**1**
• Crying steadily, screams or sobs, frequent complaints.	**2**
Consolable	
• Content, relaxed.	**0**
• Reassured by occasional touching, hugging, or being talked to; distractible.	**1**
• Difficult to console or comfort.	**2**

Referred Pain

Phenomenon of pain perceived at a site adjacent to or at a distance from site of pain's origin (e.g., cardiac pain often manifests in the arm).

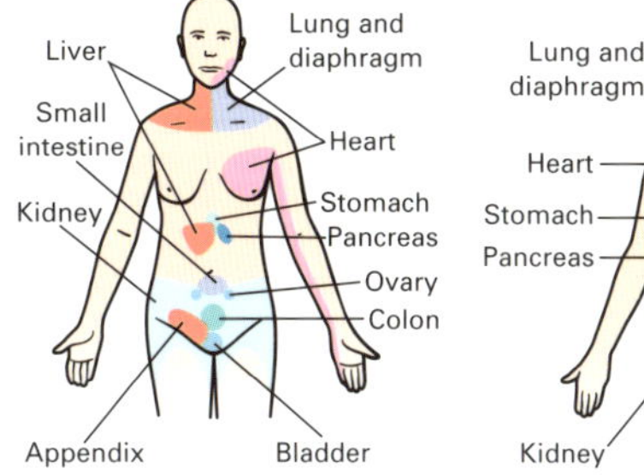

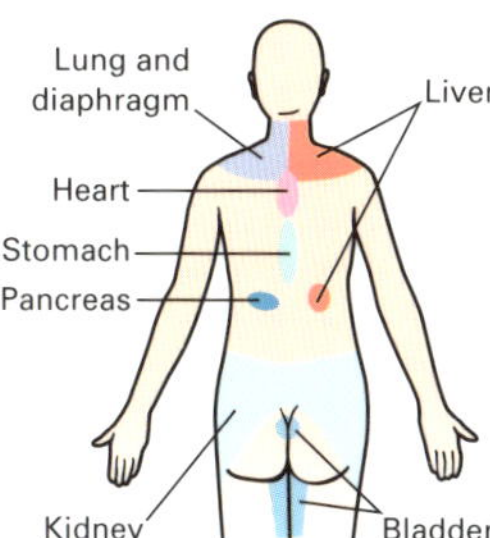

General Safety Guidelines

◎ **Be Safe!** Your safety ALWAYS comes first!

◎ **Be Aware!** Watch for nonverbal indicators of aggression or violence: clenched fists, pacing, raised tone of voice, increased respirations, profanity, verbal threats, weapons, wide-eyed stare.

◎ **Know Your Exit!** Always position yourself between Pt and an exit. Never allow Pt to block your means of escape.

◎ **Be Assertive!** Make your boundaries known, set limits, and stick to them. Avoid arguing or bargaining with Pts.

Mental Status Assessment

Appearance	Grooming, hygiene, posture, and eye contact; correlation between appearance, developmental stage, and age.
General Attitude	Cooperative, uncooperative, friendly, hostile, defensive, guarded, apathetic.
Mood	Depressed, sad, anxious, fearful, labile, irritable, elated, euphoric, guilty, despairing.
Motor Activity	Tremors, tics, mannerisms, gestures, gait, hyperactivity, restlessness, agitation, echopraxia, rigidity, aggressiveness.
Sensory/ Perceptual Disturbances	Hallucinations (auditory, visual, tactile, olfactory, gustatory) Illusions (depersonalization, derealization).
Affect	Congruent with mood, flat, inappropriate.
Cognitive	Alertness, orientation, memory, abstract thinking.
Speech Pattern	Aphasia, volume, impairments, stuttering.
Thought Process	**Form of Thought:** Tangentiality, word salads, neologisms, echolalia, attention span. **Content of Thought:** Delusional, suicidal, homicidal, obsessive, paranoid, suspicious, religiosity-based, phobic, magical.
Impulse Control	Aggression, fear, guilt, affection, sexual.
Judgment/ Insight	Decision making, problem solving, coping.

Suicidal Patient

General Guidelines

- If, at any time Pt is threatening suicide, get help. Call 911.
- Provide safe environment.
- Always take overt or covert suicide threats or attempts seriously.
- Observe Pt closely.
- Encourage expression of feelings.
- Assign tasks to increase feelings of usefulness.
- Provide full schedule of activities.
- Show acceptance, respect, and appreciation.
- Do not argue with Pt.
- Remind Pt that there are alternatives to suicide.

Groups at Increased Risk for Suicide

- Adolescent and young adult Pts (ages 15–24).
- Elderly Pts.
- Terminally ill Pts.
- Pts who have experienced stress or loss.
- Survivors of persons who have committed suicide.
- Individuals with bipolar disorder or schizophrenia.
- Pts coming out of depression.
- People who abuse alcohol or other drugs.
- Pts who have previously attempted suicide.
- More women attempt suicide; more men complete suicide.

Lethality Assessment

- **Intention:** Ask Pt if he or she thinks about and/or intends to harm self.
- **Plan:** Ask Pt if he or she has formulated a plan. What are the details: where, when, and how will plan be carried out?
- **Means:** Check availability of method: access to gun, knife, pills, etc?
- **Lethality of Means:** Pills vs. gun; jumping vs. slitting wrist.
- **Rescue:** Possibility of rescue.
- Support or lack of support.
- Anxiety or hostility level.
- Disorganized thinking.
- Preoccupation with thoughts of suicide plan.
- Prior suicide attempts.

Respiratory Assessment

History	Cough (productive or nonproductive), dyspnea, hemoptysis, CP, swelling of lower extremities, energy level, sleep pattern, COPD (asthma, chronic bronchitis, emphysema), TB, pneumonia, URI, environmental allergies.
Medication	Bronchodilators, acetylcysteine, aminophylline, theophylline, anticholinergics, corticosteroids.
Respirations	• Rate, depth, effort, pattern.
Inspect	• Signs of distress (nasal flaring or sternal retractions). • Size and shape of chest, symmetry of chest wall movement, and use of accessory muscles. • Lower extremities for edema and nail beds for cyanosis and clubbing indicating chronic hypoxia. • Trachea for scars, stomas, or deviation from midline.
Palpate	• Anterior and posterior thorax for subcutaneous emphysema, crepitus, and tenderness. • Assess tactile fremitus; palpate chest as Pt says, "99."
Percuss	• Anterior and posterior thorax for tympany (hollow organs), resonance (air-filled organs), dullness (solid organs), or flatness (muscle or bone).
Auscultate	• All anterior and posterior lung fields, noting normal, abnormal, or absence of lung sounds. • Order of auscultation: begin at the top, near the shoulders, and work toward the bottom, near the diaphragm, moving from left to right working in a zigzag pattern.

Auscultation of Lung Sounds

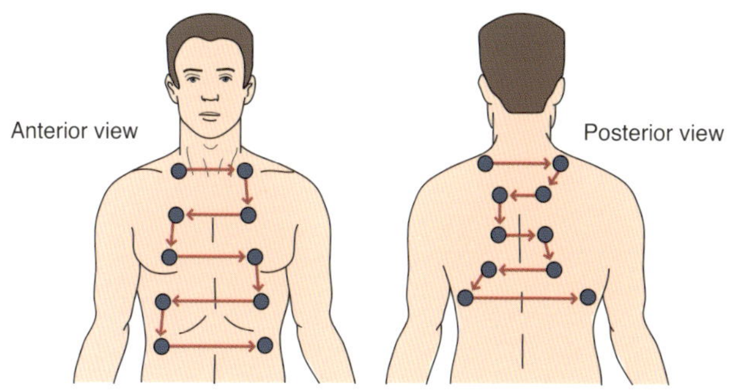

Respiratory Patterns

- **Normal (eupnea)**: Regular and comfortable at 12–20 breaths/min.
- **Tachypnea:** >20 breaths/min.
- **Bradypnea:** <12 breaths/min.
- **Hyperventilation**: Rapid, deep respiration >20 breaths/min.
- **Apneustic**: Neurological: sustained inspiratory effort
- **Cheyne Stokes**: Neurological: alternating patterns of depth separated by brief periods of apnea.
- **Kussmaul**: Rapid, deep, and labored: common in DKA.
- **Air trapping**: Difficulty during expiration: emphysema.

Lung Sounds—Differential Diagnosis

Rales/Crackles	Simulated by rolling hair near ear between two fingers, best heard on inspiration in lower bases, unrelieved by coughing, (e.g., CHF, pneumonia).
Wheezes	High-pitched, squeaking sound, best heard on expiration over all lung fields, unrelieved by coughing (e.g., asthma, COPD, emphysema).
Rhonchi	Coarse, harsh, loud gurgling or rattling, best heard on expiration over bronchi and trachea, often relieved by coughing (e.g., bronchitis, pneumonia).
Stridor	**Life-Threatening!** Harsh, high-pitched, easily audible on inspiration, progressive narrowing of upper airway requiring immediate attention (e.g., partial airway obstruction, croup, epiglottitis).
Unilaterally Absent or Diminished	Inability to hear equal, bilateral breath sounds (e.g., pneumothorax, tension pneumothorax, hemothorax, or history of pneumectomy).
Documentation	Rate, rhythm, depth, effort, sounds (indicate if sound is inspiratory and/or expiratory), and fields of auscultation.

Wound Assessment

Appearance	Color (pink, healing; yellow/green, infection; black, necrosis), sloughing, eschar, longitudinal streaking.
Size	Length, width, and depth in cm.
Incisions	Approximated edges, dehiscence, or evisceration.
Undermining	Use a sterile, cotton-tipped applicator to probe gently underneath edges until resistance is met; with a felt-tipped pen, mark where applicator can be felt under skin.
Induration	Abnormal firmness of tissues with margins. Assess by gently pinching tissue distal to wound edge; if indurated, you will be unable to pinch fold of skin.

Continued

Tissue Edema	Note whether edema is pitting or nonpitting. ◎ If wound is crepitant, notify physician immediately (may indicate gangrene).
Granulation	Bright red, shiny, and granular; an indication that wound is healing. ◎ Poorly vascularized tissue appears pale pink, dull, or dusky red.
Drainage	Type (sanguineous, serosanguineous, purulent), amount, color, and consistency.
Odor	◎ Foul odor indicates infection.
Staging	See the section that immediately follows, Areas Susceptible to Pressure Ulcers.

Areas Susceptible to Pressure Ulcers

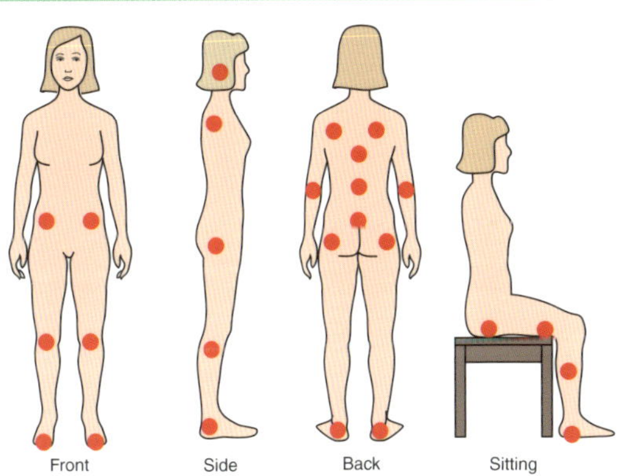

Pressure Ulcers

Stage I
- Intact, nonblanching erythematous area.
- Indicates potential for ulceration.

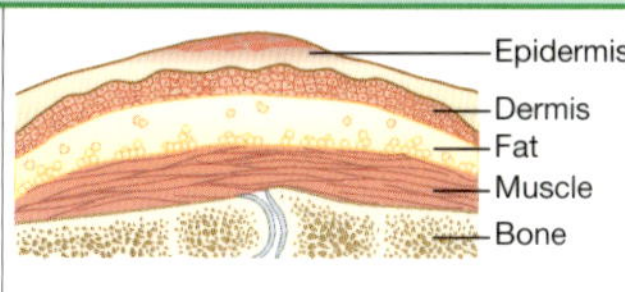

Stage II
- Interruption of epidermis, dermis, or both.
- Presents as abrasion, blister, or very shallow crater.

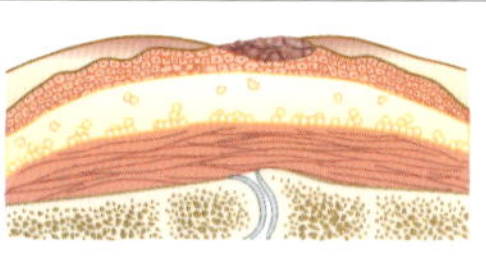

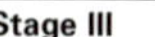

Stage III
- Full-thickness crater.
- Involves damage and/or necrosis down to, but not penetrating, fascia.

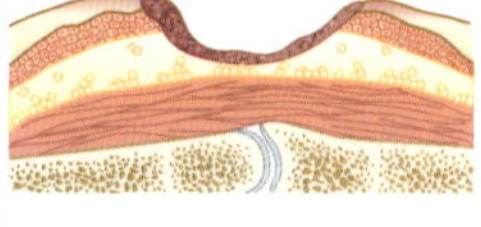

Stage IV
- Full-thickness crater.
- Similar to stage III, but penetrates fascia and involves muscle and bone.
- May involve undermining.

Pressure Ulcer Prevention Strategies

- Inspect skin at beginning of each shift and document findings. More frequent (every 2 hr) assessments are required for debilitated Pts.
- Effectively manage urine and fecal incontinence.
- Clean skin promptly with mild, nonirritating, nondrying cleaning solution, and avoid friction during cleaning.
- Use topical moisture barriers and moisture-absorbing pads if incontinent.
- Position Pts to alleviate pressure and shearing forces.
- Reposition Pts every 2 hr while in bed, and every hour while in chair.
- Teach Pt to shift weight every 15 min while in chair.
- Use appropriate positioning devices and foam padding.
- Do not use donut-shaped devices.
- Avoid positioning Pts directly on trochanters or directly on wound.
- Maintain lowest head elevation position possible to minimize sacral pressure.
- Use extra staff and appropriate lifting devices.
- Prevent contractures.
- Provide adequate hydration and nutrition.
- Do not massage reddened areas over bony prominences.

Risk Factors for Development of Pressure Ulcers

Alterations in Sensation or Response to Discomfort

- Degenerative neurological/neuromuscular disease, cerebrovascular disease, brain or spinal cord injury, depression, drugs that adversely affect alertness.

Alterations in Mobility

- Neurological disease/injury, fractures, contractures, pain, or restraints.

Significant Changes in Weight

- Protein-energy malnutrition, severe edema, obesity.

Medical Conditions

- Malnutrition and dehydration, diabetes mellitus, peripheral vascular disease, end-stage renal disease, congestive heart failure, malignant diseases, chronic obstructive pulmonary disease, obesity, or bowel and bladder incontinence.

Age-Related Changes and Implications

Physical Changes	Implication
NCLEX Decreased Skin Thickness	• Elderly Pts are more prone to skin breakdown. • Assess more frequently for pressure ulcers.
NCLEX Decreased Skin Vascularity	• Thermoregulation is altered. • Increased risk for heat stroke.
NCLEX Loss of Subcutaneous Tissue	• Insulation is decreased. • Risk for hypothermia is increased.
Decreased Aortic Elasticity	• Diastolic BP is increased.

Possible Decreased Auditory Ability	• Do not assume it, but allow for it as a possibility.
	• If Pt is hard of hearing:
	  • Approach Pt from front and make eye contact to build confidence.
	  • Speak slowly.
	  • Do not speak to Pt as if he or she were a child.

Calcification of Thoracic Wall	• Heart and lung sounds are obscured. • Apical pulse is displaced.
Loss of Nerve Fibers/ Neurons	• Extra time is needed to comprehend and learn, and to perform certain tasks
NCLEX Decreased Nerve Conduction	• Response to pain is altered.
NCLEX Reduced Tactile Sensation and Range of Motion	• Risk for injury to self is increased. • Use extra care with exams to avoid discomfort and injury.
Social Changes	**Implication**
Marital or Companion Status	Pts living alone are less likely to access health care and are more likely to suffer from heath problems, social isolation, and/or depression.
Generational Differences	**Women:** Be careful to maintain modesty when giving care. **Men:** Be careful to maintain independence when giving care.

Continued

Social Changes	Implication
Living Arrangements	Living situation affects Pt's ease of access to shopping and services, and influences available support from family and friends.
Financial Status	Income level influences Pt's ability to access health care, especially prescription drugs.
Education	Education level influences Pt's ability to understand and carry out instructions.
Caregiver Responsibilities	Pts with caregiving roles may be reluctant to report their own symptoms.
Caregiver Availability	Availability (or unavailability) of caregivers influences Pt's access to health care.
ADLs	Pts of advanced age have more difficult time completing common ADLs.
Hobbies and Interests	Lack of hobbies or interests may lead to social isolation and depression.

NCLEX Dehydration in the Elderly

Dehydration is more common in older adults and can lead to confusion, urinary and respiratory tract infections, constipation, stroke, and death.

Risk Factors

- Diminished feelings of thirst.
- Decreased total body water (TBW).
  - **Older adults:** TBW represents 60% of weight.
  - **Younger adults:** TBW represents 70% of weight.

High Risk Factors for Dehydration	
• Age >85 yr. • Nursing home resident. • Recent weight loss >5% of body weight. • Difficulties with feeding and eating, difficulty swallowing. • Dementia. • Multiple chronic conditions.	• Confinement to bed. • Polypharmacy. • Limited opportunity to drink. • Fever, vomiting, diarrhea. • Diuretic or laxative use. • Self-restriction of fluids for incontinence or increased nighttime voiding frequency.

Signs and Symptoms

- Confusion, change in LOC, dizziness.
- Tachycardia, orthostatic hypotension.
- Low urine output, dark yellow to brownish urine.
- Dry skin, poor skin turgor, dry mucous membranes.
- Constipation, fecal impaction.
- Infection, elevated temperature.
- Weakness, fatigue.
- Signs of electrolyte imbalance.
- Increased urine specific gravity.
- Increased hematocrit.

Nursing Interventions

◎ Notify physician or charge nurse immediately if signs or symptoms of dehydration are present.

◎ Dehydration can progress quickly and become severe, and it is associated with a high mortality rate in elderly Pts.

- Evaluate hydration status by assessing:
  - Vital signs
  - Urine specific gravity
  - Complete blood count
  - Urine color
  - 24-hr fluid I&O
  - NPO status
  - Enteral/tube feedings
  - Usual pattern of fluid intake

Calculating Desired Fluid Intake Per Day	
Start with Pt's Weight (kg)	**Example if Pt Weighs 70 kg**
Subtract 20	= 50
Multiply by 15	= 750
Add 1500	= 2250
Multiply by 0.75	= 1688 mL/day (desired intake)

- Provide 80% of desired fluid goal at meals.
- Provide remaining 20% between meals.
- Offer various fluids and have Pt take sips throughout day if he or she has trouble taking more at one time.
- Document I&O and difficulty drinking.

- Assess weight daily and record.
- Note urine specific gravity and urine color.
- Post volume of each container (e.g., cups, bowls) in Pt's room.
- For test preparation (NPO or bowel cleansing), arrange timing so that test occurs as soon as possible. Offer fluids immediately after test unless contraindicated. Consider IV hydration if NPO status is prolonged.

Delirium and Dementia in the Elderly

- **Delirium:** Confusion/excitement marked by disorientation to time and place, usually accompanied by delusions and/or hallucinations.
- **Dementia:** Cognitive deficits.
- **Depression:** Diminished interest or pleasure in most or all activities.

Factor	Delirium	Dementia
Onset	Sudden	Gradual
Duration	Brief (hours–days)	Long (months–years)
LOC	Fluctuating throughout day	Unaffected
Motor	Tremor, myoclonus, ataxia, hyperactivity	None until late
Speech	Incoherent	Normal to aphasic in later stages
Language	Vocabulary usual for Pt, but frequent use of wrong words	Impoverished, worsens as disorder progresses
Memory	Impaired	Impaired
Attention	Impaired, fluctuating	Normal to easily distracted
Perception	Hallucinations common	Hallucinations uncommon
Mood	Fearful, suspicious, irritable	Fearful, suspicious, irritable, normal affect, depressed early in disorder
Sleep	Disturbances common	Disturbances common
General Condition	Sick appearing	Healthy appearing
Clinical Course	Fluctuating over short term	Stable over short term

Depression and Suicide in the Elderly

Depression is common in older adults, is often unreported and unrecognized, diminishes quality of life, and can lead to suicide.

Physical

- Pain, stomach problems.
- Changes in appetite.
- Feeling tired all the time.
- Insomnia or excessive sleeping.

Emotional

- Unrelenting sadness.
- Diminished pleasure.
- Crying for no reason.
- Indifference to others.
- Feeling hopeless, helpless, and worthless.

Cognitive

- Impaired concentration.
- Problems with memory.
- Indecisiveness.
- Recurrent thoughts of death and suicide.

Behavioral

- Neglect of personal appearance; hygiene.
- Withdrawal from others.
- Increased alcohol use.
- Agitation; anxiety.

Signs of Suicidal Intent

- Talking about death as relief.
- Giving away possessions.
- Stopping medication.
- Obtaining a weapon.

Nursing Interventions

- Assess Pt for signs and symptoms of depression.
- Ask whether he or she has thought about committing suicide.
- Show interest and offer support; talking can help older adults identify main themes of their lives, express regret, and talk about their legacy.
- Avoid giving advice or conversation altogether—just listen.
- Identify Pt's support among friends, family, and clergy.
- Remove implements or meds that can be used for suicide.
- Notify staff, document findings, and participate in plan of care.

Eating Problems in the Elderly

Possible Causes	Nursing Interventions
GI Disturbances • Difficulty swallowing. • Constipation. • Nausea and vomiting. • Gastric reflux (GERD).	• Observe Pt for signs of swallowing difficulty (coughing while eating, holding food in mouth, frequently attempting to clear throat); consult with speech therapist. • Monitor bowel patterns or any trouble passing stool; assess for impaction. • Investigate cause of nausea and vomiting, and assess for symptoms of GERD.
Oral Problems • Missing or poorly fitting dentures. • Missing teeth, dental cavities, gum disease. • Dry mouth.	• Inspect dentures for proper fit, use dental adhesive, and consider dental consult. • Provide oral care before and after meals. • Offer fluids frequently during meals to provide sufficient moisture to chew and swallow foods.
Functional Deficits • Weakness; inability to feed self; tremors. • Difficulty sitting, confinement to bed. • Poor vision, less discriminating taste buds, and other sensory deficits.	• Suggest consultation with OT for assistive devices. • If Pt needs to be fed, offer small spoonfuls and allow ample time for chewing/swallowing. • Ensure Pt is in upright position for eating. • Use assistive devices including glasses, hearing aids, and specially handled utensils.
Neurological Issues • Depression. • Anxiety. • Pain. • Dementia.	• Work with health-care team to manage pain, anxiety, and/or depression effectively. • Provide consistent staff members to feed Pt; have family member present at mealtimes, if possible.
Medication Side Effects • Anorexia. • Nausea, vomiting. • Taste changes. • Constipation. • Drowsiness.	• Evaluate meds for possible source. • Work with health-care team to change or discontinue drugs, if possible. • Treat adverse effects if meds cannot be changed (e.g., antiemetics). • Evaluate effects of interventions.

Fall Risk Assessment and Prevention

Risk Factor	Intervention
Assessment Data • Age >65 yr. • History of falls.	• Monitor frequently. • Pt should be close to nurses' station. • Implement fall prevention interventions.
Medications • Polypharmacy. • CNS depressants. • BP/HR lowering. • Diuretics. • GI motility meds.	• Review meds with physician. • Assess for meds that may affect BP, HR, balance, or LOC. • Educate about use of sedatives, narcotics, and vasoactive meds. • Encourage nonopioid pain management.
Mental Status • Altered LOC or orientation.	• Routinely reorient Pt to situation. • Maintain a structured environment. • Use pressure-sensitive bed/chair alarms.
Cardiovascular • Postural hypotension.	• Change positions slowly. • Review MAR for possible changes.
Neurosensory • Visual impairment. • Peripheral neuropathy. • Difficulty with balance or gait.	• Provide illumination at night. • Minimize clutter and remove unnecessary equipment from room. • Provide protective footwear. • Provide appropriate assistive devices and instruct on proper use.
GI/GU • Incontinence. • Urinary frequency. • Diarrhea.	• Ensure call light is within easy reach. • Create toileting schedule. • Provide bedside commode or urinal or unobstructed, well-lit path to bathroom.
Musculoskeletal • Decreased range of motion. • Amputee.	• Provide range-of-motion exercises and stretching. • Provide PT or OT consults. • Provide appropriate assistive devices.
Assistive Devices • Use of cane, walker, or WC.	• Ensure that assistive devices are not damaged and are appropriately sized. • Instruct Pt on proper and safe use.
Environment • Cluttered room. • Tubes and lines.	• Minimize clutter; remove unnecessary or infrequently used equipment. • Ensure call light is within easy reach.

Fall Prevention

Skilled Nursing Facility

- Identify and report unsafe conditions.
- Avoid excessive use of sedatives.
- Refer unsteady Pts to PT or OT.
- Teach the correct use of assistive devices.
- Review medication record.
- Emphasize need to change body position gradually.
- Encourage strength and range-of-motion exercises.
- Teach about appropriate attire (e.g., sturdy shoes).
- Inform provider of recent changes in hearing, vision, or physical abilities.
- Notify provider of untoward effects of meds.

At Home

- Arrange furniture to ensure unobstructed pathway.
- Keep all pathways well-lit.
- Install lights and light switches at top and bottom of stairs.
- Ensure excess cords are coiled and next to wall.
- Avoid using throw rugs.
- Fix uneven or damaged steps, and install handrails on both sides of entire length of stairs.
- Use steady step stool with grip bar and keep often used items at waist level.
- Install grab bars in tub and in bathroom next to toilet.
- Ensure nonslip surfaces in bathroom floor and tub.

Pharmacokinetics in the Elderly

Definition: Pharmacokinetics is the way the body absorbs, distributes, metabolizes, and excretes medication.

⊚ Age-related physiological changes affect body systems, alter pharmacokinetics, and increase or alter a drug's effect.

	Physiological Change	Effect on Pharmacokinetics
Absorption	• Decreased intestinal motility. • Diminished blood flow to gut.	• Delayed peak effect. • Delayed signs and symptoms of toxicity.
Distribution	• Decreased fluid volume.	• Increased serum concentration of water-soluble drugs.
	• Increased body fat percentage.	• Increased half-life of fat-soluble drugs.
	• Decreased plasma proteins.	• Increased amount of active drug.
	• Decreased lean body mass.	• Increased drug concentration.
Metabolism	• Decreased blood flow to liver.	• Decreased rate of drug clearance by liver.
	• Decreased liver function.	• Increased accumulation of some drugs.
Excretion	• Decreased kidney function. • Decreased creatinine clearance.	• Increased accumulation of drugs normally excreted by kidneys.

Polypharmacy in the Elderly

Definition: Polypharmacy is concurrent use of several drugs. Taking two drugs increases risk of an adverse drug event by 6%.

◎ Taking eight drugs increases risk of an adverse drug event by 100%.

Assessment and Prevention

- Have pharmacy and physician regularly review meds.
- Take complete medication history, including OTC and herbal supplements.
- Evaluate all meds for correct dose, duplication, and potential for drug–drug interactions; look up contraindications.
- Coordinate care if Pt has multiple physicians.
- Educate Pt and family about medication use.
- Encourage Pts to use one pharmacy for all their prescriptions.
- Help Pts develop simple medication regimen.
- Ensure that all pill bottles are easy to read and are labeled correctly.
- Encourage nonpharmacological treatments whenever possible.

OB Patients: Pregnancy—Newborn—Postpartum

Basic Terms Associated With Pregnancy

Abortion	Spontaneous or induced termination of pregnancy before fetus reaches viability
Chloasma	Mask of pregnancy
Crowning	Presentation of fetal head at vaginal introitus
CST	Contraction stress test
Deceleration	Decrease in fetal heart rate
Dilation	Widening of cervical os and canal
Eclampsia	Seizures secondary to hypertension
EDD or EDC	Estimated date of delivery or confinement
Embryo phase	Wk 3–8
Effacement	Shortening and thinning of cervix
Fetus phase	From wk 9 until delivery
FHR	Fetal heart rate
FHT	Fetal heart tone
Gravida	Number of all pregnancies, regardless of outcome, including current pregnancy (gravidity)
GTPAL	Gravidity, term births, preterm births, abortions or miscarriages, living children

HELLP . . . . .Hemolysis, elevated liver enzymes, lowered platelets (bleeding disorder similar to DIC)
Homans' sign . . . . .Pain elicited by dorsiflexion of foot
Hyperemesis gravidarum . . . . . .Excessive nausea and vomiting in early pregnancy
IDM . . . . .Infant of diabetic mother
Involution .Return of uterus to nonpregnant size
Lanugo . . . . .Soft, downy body hair of newborn infant
LGA . . . . .Large for gestational age
LNMP (LMP) . . . . .Last normal menstrual period
L:S ratio . . . . .Lecithin/sphingomyelin ratio: determines fetal lung maturity (2:1 ratio desirable)
MAb . . . . .Miscarriage abortion
Macrosomia . . . . .Birth weight >4000 g
Meconium .Fetal defecation in utero during labor that occurs with fetal distress
Miscarriage . . . . .Spontaneous abortion
Multigravida . . . . .Has been pregnant more than once
Multipara .Two or more pregnancies beyond 20 wk
Nidation . . . . .Implantation: occurs 7–10 days after conception
NST . . . . .Nonstress test
Nullipara . . . . .Never produced a viable offspring
OCT . . . . .Oxytocin challenge test
Operculum . . . . .Mucous plug
Organogenesis . . . . .Wk 3–8
Para . . . . .Number of viable births >20 wk (parity)
Pica . . . . .Ingestion of non-nutritive substances
PIH . . . . .Pregnancy-induced hypertension (see pre-eclampsia this section)
Post-term .Gestation lasting >42 wk
POC . . . . .Product of conception
Pre-eclampsia . . . . .Mild: ≥140/90 mm Hg; severe: ≥160/110 mm Hg
Pre-term . . . . .Born before beginning of 38th wk
Primigravida . . . . .First pregnancy ever
Primipara .Only one pregnancy carried >20 wk
PTL . . . . .Preterm labor
Puerperal period . . . .≤21–42 days postpartum
ROM . . . . .Rupture of membranes (1000 mL at term)
SGA . . . . .Small for gestational age
Station, fetal . . . . .Relation of presenting part to maternal pelvic ischial spines
Striae . . . . .Stretch marks
Supine hypotension . . . . .Caused by compression of vena cava; relieved by positioning mother in lateral recumbent position

TAb . . . . .Therapeutic abortion
Teratogenic . . . . .Harmful to developing embryo
TPAL .Term, preterm births, abortions or miscarriages, living children
Trimester . . . . .One of three phases of pregnancy, each consisting of 13 wk
Variability . . . . .Refers to irregularities in fetal heart rate
Vernix . . . . .Cheeselike coating on newborn's skin
Viability . . . . .Pregnancy lasting beyond 20 wk of gestation
Viable fetus . . . . .Uncompromised fetus beyond 20 wk

Due Date Prediction (Nägele's Rule)

1. **Add 7 days to first day of LMP**: LMP 7/14/07 + 7 = 7/21/07.
2. **Subtract 3 months:** 7/21/07 – 3 months = 4/21/07.
3. **Add 1 year:** 4/21/07 + 1 year = 4/21/08 (EDD).

Fetal Development Timetable

4 wk	0.4 cm, 0.4 g	**24 wk**	28 cm, 780 g
8 wk	3 cm, 2 g	**28 wk**	38 cm, 1200 g
12 wk	8 cm, 19 g	**32 wk**	40 cm, 2000 g
16 wk	12.5 cm, 100 g	**36 wk**	42 cm, 2500 g
20 wk	19 cm, 465 g	**40 wk**	50 cm, 3200 g

Fundal Height Assessment

- Fundal height is measured to assess fetal growth and development.
- Using cm ruler, measure from top of symphysis pubis to top of fundus (subtract 1 cm if pt is very obese).
- Measurements >4 cm from estimated gestational age require further evaluation.

Gestation (wk)	12	16	20	24	28	32	36	40
Height (cm)	11–13	15–17	19–21	23–24	27–29	31–33	35–37	33–35

Hormones Associated With Pregnancy

- **Follicle-stimulating hormone (FSH)**: Follicle growth and maturation
- **Luteinizing hormone (LH)**: Egg development and ovulation
- **Progesterone**: Maintenance of pregnancy
- **Prolactin**: Initiation and continuation of milk production (lactation)
- **Oxytocin**: Stimulation of uterine contractions and milk letdown

Immunization During Pregnancy: 2013

Recommended

◎ For persons who meet age requirement and who lack evidence of immunity (e.g., documentation).

- Tetanus, diphtheria, pertussis (Td/Tdap)
- Influenza (one dose TIV annually)

Recommended

◎ Only if medical or exposure indication exists.

- Pneumococcal
- Hepatitis A
- Hepatitis B
- Meningococcal

Contraindicated During Pregnancy

- Varicella
- Zoster
- MMR (measles, mumps, rubella)

Source: Centers for Disease Control and Prevention, U.S. Department of Health and Human Services, 2011 recommendations; http://www.cdc.gov/vaccines/schedules/downloads/adult/adult-schedule-easy-read.pdf.

Normal Changes Throughout Pregnancy

Cardiovascular

- HR . . . . . Increases
- BP . . . . . Lower first half, no change last half
- Blood volume . . . . . ≤50% increase
- Hgb and Hct . . . . . Decrease
- RBC . . . . . ≤30% increase
- WBC . . . . . Increases
- Vasodilation . . . . . Caused by increased progesterone levels

- Stroke volume . . . . .Increases
- CO . . . . .Increases
- SVR . . . . .Decreases
- Supine position . . . . .Decreases perfusion to fetus

Respiratory

- Respiratory rate . . . . .Increases
- Oxygen consumption . . . . .Increases by 15%
- Tidal volume . . . . .Increases
- Functional residual capacity . . . . .Decreases
- Dyspnea . . . . .Normal at end of third trimester
- pH . . . . .Increases
- PaO_2 . . . . .Increases
- $PaCO_2$ . . . . .Decreases
- HCO_3 . . . . .Decreases

Renal

- Proteinuria . . . . .May indicate possible PIH
- GFR . . . . .Increases by ≤50%

Metabolic

- Temperature . . . . .Slightly increases
- Blood glucose . . . . .Increase may indicate gestational diabetes

Weight Gain and Nutritional Requirements

Optimal Weight Gain

- NCLEX Total weight gain during pregnancy .25–35 lb
- First trimester . . . .~2–3 lb
- Second–third trimester . . . . .3/4 lb every wk

Nutritional Requirements

- NCLEX Additional caloric needs . . . . .300 cal/day (2500 total)
- Protein . . . . .75 g/day
- Carbohydrates . . . . .175 g/day (mostly complex)
- Fiber . . . . .28 g/day
- Fats . . . . .20–35 g/day
- Sodium . . . . . . .Should not be restricted unless under physician's guidance
- Iron . . . . .27 mg/day
- Calcium . . . . .1000 mg/day
- Folic acid .600 mcg/day (500 mcg/day while lactating)
- Daily fluid intake . . . .~3 L/day unless pre-eclampsia exists

Progression of Labor

Factors Affecting Progression of Labor (Four Ps)

- **Passenger:** Size of fetus and its head, fetal presentation, lie, attitude, and position in relation to birth canal.
- **Passageway:** Size of birth canal in relation to fetus.
- **Power:** Force, regularity, and duration of contractions.
- **Psychological:** Pain and anxiety experienced by mother, including preparation for delivery and support system.

NCLEX Stages of Labor

Stage I	From onset of contractions through full effacement and dilation of cervix (latent phase, 0–3 cm; active phase, 4–7 cm; transition phase, 8–10 cm); duration: 8–18 hr.
Stage II	From full dilation of cervix until delivery of baby; duration: 15–90 min.
Stage III	From birth of baby until expulsion of placenta; duration: ≤20 min.
Stage IV	First 1–4 hr after expulsion of placenta.

Comparison of True and False Labor

	True Labor	False Labor
Contractions	Consistent pattern	Inconsistent pattern
Frequency of Contractions	Progressively increasing	Inconsistent
Duration of Contractions	Progressively increasing	Inconsistent
Intensity of Contractions	Progressively increasing; increases with walking	Inconsistent; subsides or does not increase with walking
Cervix	Progressive effacement and dilation	No significant change
Discomfort	Mostly low back and abdominal	Mostly abdominal and groin

Electronic Fetal Monitoring

Fetal Heart Rate (FHR)

- **Normal:** 120–160 bpm (can be higher for short periods, <10 min).
- **Tachycardia:** Sustained FHR >160 for >10 min; common causative factor can include early fetal hypoxia, immaturity, amnionitis, maternal fever, and terbutaline.
- **Bradycardia:** Sustained FHR <120 for >10 min; common causative factor can include late or profound fetal hypoxia, maternal hypotension, prolonged umbilical cord compression, and anesthetics.

Fetal Heart Rate Patterns

Reassuring (normal) Pattern

- Baseline FHR 130–140 bpm; preserved beat to beat.
- Long-term variability.
- Accelerations last ≥15 sec above baseline.
- Accelerations peak at ≥15 bpm.

Early Decelerations

- Mirror image of contraction.
- Starts and stops with contractions.
- **Etiology:** Head compression.
- **Management:** Observation.

Variable Pattern

- Occurs at unpredictable times during contractions.
- Size and shape vary.
- **Etiology:** Cord compression.
- **Management:** Lateral position, oxygen, c-section if not corrected.

Late Decelerations

- Reverse mirror image of contractions.
- Starts after contraction begins; stops after contraction ends.
- **Etiology:** Uteroplacental insufficiency.
- **Management:** Lateral position, stop or slow pitocin, oxygen, IV fluids, c-section if not corrected.

Variability (Cardiac Rhythm Irregularities)

- **None:** 0–2 variations/min (abnormal).
- **Minimal:** 3–5 variations/min (abnormal).
- **Average:** 6–10 variations/min (normal).
- **Moderate:** 11–25 variations/min (normal).
- **Marked:** >25 variations/min (abnormal).

EARLY DECELERATION

Cause: Fetal head compression (HC)

Example:

Uniform Shape
180
FHR
100
Early onset
50
UC
0

LATE DECELERATION

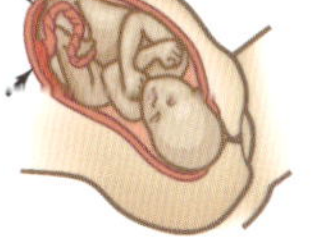

Cause: Uteroplacental insufficiency (UPI)

Example:

Uniform shape
180
FHR
100
Late onset
1 min.
50
UC
0

VARIABLE DECELERATION

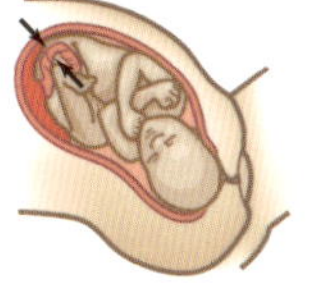

Cause: Umbilical cord compression (CC)

Example:

Variable shape
180
FHR
100
Variable onset
50
UC
0

Complications of Pregnancy

NCLEX Bleeding: Placenta Abruptio

Definition: Premature separation of placenta from uterine wall.
Incidence: Occurring in approximately 1 in 120 deliveries and more likely to affect multipara women and women older than 35 yr.
Onset: May occur during prenatal or intrapartum period.
Etiology: Unknown; pre-eclampsia and HTN possible causes.
Symptoms: Dark red vaginal bleeding (may be concealed), severe tearing sensation, abdominal and lower back pain, signs of shock.

Four Grades of Abruptio

Grade 0: <10% detachment, mother and fetus asymptomatic, small retroplacental clot noted at birth.
Grade I: 10%–20% detachment, mild bleeding and uterine tenderness, mother and fetus not in distress.
Grade II: 20%–50% detachment, uterine tenderness and tetany, signs of fetal distress noted, but mother not in hypovolemic shock.
Grade III: >50% detachment, severe uterine tenderness and tetany, hemorrhage, shock, and fetal death; coagulopathy (HELLP syndrome) likely to occur.

Collaborative Care

- Continuous internal fetal monitoring is performed for signs of distress.
- Supplemental oxygen is administered and IV access is established.
- Labs include CBC, coagulation studies, and type and crossmatch.
- Vaginal delivery is permitted if mother and fetus are not in any distress.
- Emergency c-section is performed if mother and fetus are in distress.
- Blood transfusion may be given for excessive hemorrhage.
- If mother and fetus are stable and pregnancy is <28 wk along, mother is discharged home on tocolytic medications (to inhibit uterine contractions).
- Position Pt on left side if fetus is showing signs of distress.
- Vital signs and mother are monitored closely for signs of shock.
- Assess for signs of occult bleeding: rigid, boardlike abdomen, constant abdominal pain, increased fundal height, late decelerations, or decreased variability of FHR.

Reinforce Patient Teaching

- Provide Pt and family with literature on placenta abruptio.
- Instruct Pt to notify physician of any cramping or bleeding.
- Explain actions, dosages, side effects, and adverse reactions of meds.

NCLEX Bleeding: Placenta Previa

Definition: Implantation of placenta in lower segment of uterus that causes partial or complete coverage of cervical os.

Incidence: Approximately 1 in 200 term deliveries and more likely to affect multipara women and women older than 35 yr.

Onset: Bleeding often occurring as early as 28 wk, but possibly not until onset of labor, depending on type of placenta previa.

Etiology: Unknown.

Symptoms: Painless, bright red bleeding, usually after wk 28.

Four Types of Placenta Previa

Low-lying: Implantation in lower uterine segment, but not reaching cervical os; usually without associated complications.

Marginal: Edge of placenta at edge of internal os; mother possibly able to deliver vaginally.

Partial: Partial coverage of cervical os; bleeding during dilation and effacement; c-section usually required.

Total: Total coverage of cervical os; emergency c-section usually required.

Collaborative Care

- Maintenance IV, bedrest, and electronic fetal monitoring are indicated.
- For fetal distress, mother is placed in left lateral position; administer high-flow oxygen, IV fluids, and notify physician stat.
- Once bleeding has ceased for >24–48 hr, and neither mother nor fetus is in any distress, Pt may be discharged to home and put on bedrest.
- Monitor mother's vital signs and fetus for any signs of distress (variability, late decelerations, increase or decrease in HR).
- Monitor for bleeding and note amount and character of blood loss.
- Continue monitoring for signs of hypovolemic shock.
- Maintain bedrest in left lateral position to enhance venous return and perfusion to placenta.

Reinforce Patient Teaching

- Provide Pt and family with literature on placenta previa.
- If Pt is discharged before delivery, instruct her to notify her physician immediately for any vaginal bleeding, decreased fetal activity, spontaneous rupture of membranes, or contractions.
- Stress importance and benefits of lying in left lateral position.
- Instruct Pt to abstain from sexual intercourse.

NCLEX BLEEDING: PLACENTA ABRUPTIO VERSUS PLACENTA PREVIA

	Placenta Abruptio	Placenta Previa
Onset	May occur during prenatal or intrapartum period.	Bleeding often occurs as early as 28 wk, but possibly not until onset of labor.
Neuro	Anxiety, fear, restlessness.	Anxiety, fear, restlessness.
Resp	Tachypnea if in shock.	Usually unremarkable.
CV	Signs of shock.	May exhibit shock.
Skin	Cool, pale, diaphoretic.	Usually unremarkable.
GI/GU	**Dark red vaginal bleeding.** Bleeding possibly concealed, depending on grade of abruptio.	**Painless, bright red bleeding.**
MS (Pain)	**Severe tearing sensation,** abdominal and low back.	Usually unremarkable.

NCLEX Blood Pressure (Elevated): Pre-eclampsia

Definition: Multisystem disorder of pregnancy characterized by classic triad of symptoms: hypertension, proteinuria, and edema.

Incidence: 7% of all pregnancies and more likely to affect pregnant adolescents and women >35 yr.

Onset: Wk 20 and continuing throughout pregnancy, throughout labor, and ≤6 wk postpartum.

Etiology: Unknown.

Symptoms: HTN, edema, proteinuria, hyperreflexia, clonus, headache, visual disturbances, vasospasm, decreased UO, seizures.

Mild Pre-eclampsia	Severe Pre-eclampsia
• BP >140/90 and <110/160 mm Hg • 1+ to 2+ protein in urine • Protein <5 g/24 hr urine	• BP >110/160 mm Hg • 3+ to 4+ protein in urine • Protein >5 g/24 hr urine

- In mild cases, mother is treated at home on bedrest with education about warning signs and need for frequent prenatal visits.
- In moderate-to-severe cases, mother is hospitalized on complete bedrest for continuous monitoring and management.
- IV infusion of magnesium may be started to prevent seizures.
- Glucocorticoid steroids may be given IM 48 hr before delivery to assist in maturing fetal lung development.
- C-section is preformed if pre-eclampsia is severe and not responding to treatment or if fetus shows signs of distress.

Nursing Focus

- Maintain Pt on bedrest in left lateral position.
- Reduce environmental stimuli, and encourage rest.
- Keep bed in lowest position, side rails up and covered with pads.
- Assess VS, daily weight, I&O, UO, labs, and neurological status.
- Assess edema, deep tendon reflexes, and presence of clonus.
- During labor, monitor FHR and contractions, and monitor for seizures.

Reinforce Patient Teaching

- Provide Pt and family with literature on pre-eclampsia.
- Stress importance and benefits of lying in left lateral position.
- ◎ If Pt to be treated at home, instruct her to notify nurse or physician immediately for any of the following symptoms: headache, visual disturbances, sudden weight gain, altered mental status, decreased UO, RUQ pain, facial edema, or decreased fetal activity.

NCLEX Blood Pressure (Low): Supine Hypotensive Syndrome

Definition: When a pregnant woman lies on her back, the heavy gravid uterus compresses the IVC and results in pooling of blood in legs, decreased venous return, a decline in CO, and hypotension.

Onset: Becomes more pronounced as pregnancy progresses.

Neurological: Dizziness, syncope, fatigue.

CV: Hypotension, tachycardia.

Skin: Pallor, diaphoresis.

GI/GU: Nausea.

Nursing Focus

- Position mother on left side to relieve compression of IVC, and enhance venous return and uteroplacental perfusion.
- Monitor vital signs.

Reinforce Patient Teaching

- Provide Pt and family with literature on supine hypotensive syndrome.
- Stress importance and benefits of lying in left lateral position.

Gestational Diabetes

Definition: Maternal hyperglycemia (insulin resistance that begins or is first diagnosed during pregnancy).
Incidence: Approximately 4% of all pregnancies.
Onset: Usually between 24th and 28th wk of pregnancy.
Etiology: Placental hormones (estrogen, cortisol, and human placental lactogen) make cells more resistant to insulin; risk factors include a history of DM, obesity, and >35 yr.
Symptoms: Polydipsia, polyuria, polyphagia, weight loss, fatigue, nausea, vomiting, frequent infections, blurred vision.

Complications

- **Neonatal hypoglycemia:** Caused by a sudden drop in glucose, once supplied by mother, coupled with continuation of insulin production. Infants must be monitored and treated aggressively.
- **Macrosomia:** Caused by excess insulin secreted by fetus in response to elevated maternal blood glucose levels. Excess insulin acts like a growth hormone and results in a fetus that is >4500 g (LGA). C-section may be required.

Collaborative Care

- Goal of treatment is to maintain blood glucose levels within normal limits (70–105 mg/dL) during pregnancy.
- Frequent prenatal visits are indicated to monitor maternal blood glucose levels.
- Fetal growth and development are monitored using ultrasound and NSTs to measure movement and FHR variations.
- Dietary modifications and an exercise program are prescribed.
- If dietary management fails, mother may be started on SC insulin.
- Obtain and document blood glucose levels at prenatal visits.
- Assess and document fetal development (e.g., fundal height).

Reinforce Patient Teaching

- Provide Pt and family with literature on gestational diabetes.
- Encourage dietary modifications including foods high in nutrition and low in fat and calories such as fruits, vegetables, and whole grains, and stress importance of avoiding refined sugars.
- Encourage aerobic activity (30–45 min most days of the week).
- Explain actions, dosages, side effects, and adverse reactions of meds.

Hyperemesis Gravidarum

Definition: Intractable nausea and vomiting during first trimester that adversely affects nutrition and causes fluid and electrolyte imbalances.
Onset: Anytime during pregnancy.
Neuro: Fatigue, malaise.
CV: Hypotension, tachycardia.
F and E: Dehydration, electrolyte imbalances.
GI/GU: Nausea and vomiting.

Collaborative Care

- Antiemetics are prescribed.
- IV fluids may be administered for dehydration or electrolyte imbalance.
- In severe cases, total parenteral nutrition may be required.

Nursing Focus

- Place mother in position of comfort, ideally on left side to relieve compression of IVC and enhance venous return and uteroplacental perfusion.
- Monitor labs and I&O for signs of dehydration, malnourishment, and electrolyte imbalance.
- Implement fetal monitoring (e.g., FHR, activity) as ordered.

Reinforce Patient Teaching

- Provide Pt and family with literature on hyperemesis gravidum.
- Stress importance and benefits of eating small, frequent meals consisting of limited fat and easily digestible carbohydrates.
- Avoid lying flat too soon after eating, and drink liquids between meals.

Delivery—Uncomplicated

◎ Be familiar with location of emergency delivery kit and equipment.

◎ Always don gloves when imminent delivery is suspected.

Clinical Findings (Imminent Delivery)

- Contractions usually regular, <2 min apart, and progressively increasing in frequency and duration.
- Low back and abdominal pain and/or cramping.
- Mother sitting on one buttock.
- Urge to have bowel movement or strong urge to push.
- Bulging vaginal opening or crowning of baby's head.
- Mother grunting with respirations.

Assisting During Delivery

- Assess contractions (regularity, duration, and frequency).
- **If birth not imminent:** Encourage Pt to take slow, deep breaths during contractions; discourage pushing between contractions.
- **If birth imminent:** Encourage Pt to push during contractions.
- **Head:** As head delivers, examine neck for looped cord and gently slip it over baby's head if present; applying gentle pressure against baby's head during delivery will help to prevent an explosive delivery and tearing of perineum.
- Be prepared to assist with suctioning: mouth first, then nose, before next contraction (tear away amniotic sac if covering face).
- **Shoulders:** Position hands on either side of baby's head and (1) gently guide baby downward until upper shoulder emerges, then (2) guide baby upward as body emerges.
- Keep baby at same level as perineum until cord is cut.
- Hypothermia can occur rapidly in newborns; dry and wrap newborn's body and head (not face) in dry, warm blankets.
- Reassess airway, and suction mouth and nose as needed.
- Stimulate respirations with vigorous rubbing and drying.
- **Cord:** Assist in clamping the cord at 8 and 10 in. from newborn.
- Position baby (skin to skin) on mother's abdomen or chest.
- Do not pull on umbilical cord if placenta has not delivered.
- Encourage breastfeeding or massage mother's abdomen to stimulate uterine contractions.
- **Assess cord vessels:** Normally three vessels (one vein, two arteries).
- Document APGAR score at 1 and 5 min postpartum.
- Assess for postpartum complications (e.g., hemorrhage).

Delivery—With Complications

Breech Presentation

Buttocks First

- If baby has delivered to level of umbilicus, gently extract baby's legs.
- Gently extract enough cord to relieve tension on cord during delivery.

Both Feet First

- Support baby's legs and buttocks, and gently pull during contractions until shoulders are delivered.
- Avoid pulling on baby once shoulders have delivered.
- Place gloved fingers between baby's face and vaginal wall to create an airway for baby until head delivers.
- Prepare for emergency c-section

NCLEX Cord Presentation (Prolapsed Cord)

- Place mother in Trendelenburg position (left-lateral if birth not imminent).
- Relieve cord pressure with gentle pressure to baby's head.
- Monitor cord pulses and cover with saline-soaked gauze.
- Do not attempt to push cord back into uterus.
- Discourage mother from pushing during contractions to minimize cord pressure (panting instead will help to avoid pushing).
- Prepare for emergency c-section.

Limb Presentation

- Place mother in Trendelenburg position to slow delivery.
- Support presenting limb and assess pulse if possible.
- Discourage mother from pushing during contractions (panting instead will help to avoid pushing).
- Prepare for emergency c-section.

Meconium-Stained Amniotic Fluid

During Delivery

- Suction mouth first, then nose, with a bulb syringe before delivery of shoulders to prevent aspiration of meconium.

After Delivery

- If newborn is not vigorous, minimize stimulation and delay ventilation until meconium can be suctioned from airway.

If Newborn Is Depressed (HR <100, Depressed RR/muscle tone)

- Intubate newborn's trachea, but DO NOT ventilate.
- Apply suction and withdraw ET tube to clear meconium.
- Repeat process until no further meconium can be suctioned.
- During process, administer 100% O_2 via blowby.
- Ventilate newborn using bag-valve device after suctioning.

Vaginal Bleeding

Do not perform vaginal exam or attempt vaginal packing.

Antepartum (Before Delivery)

- Apply perineal pad; note time to assess amount of bleeding.
- Position mother on left side! Relieves compression of IVC and enhances venous return and uteroplacental perfusion.
- Prepare for emergency c-section if necessary.

NCLEX Postpartum Hemorrhage

Massage mother's fundus (abdomen) or encourage breastfeeding if appropriate to stimulate uterine contractions.

Control external bleeding with direct (external) pressure.

Place mother in Trendelenburg position.

Establish 2nd large-bore IV and titrate to SBP >90 mm Hg.

Oxytocin may be prescribed: (postpartum hemorrhage only!) 10 units mixed in 1000 mL LR titrated to effect (give 3–10 units IM if no IV access).

Newborn—Cardiopulmonary Resuscitation

Assessment and Stabilization

30 sec	Term gestation; HR >100; breathing or crying; good muscle tone; good RR and effort; no cyanosis	→	Keep with mother; routine care; dry, keep warm; reposition prn; clear airway prn; ongoing assessment
	Preterm (<38 weeks); poor muscle tone; not crying	→	Dry, warm, O_2 prn; clear airway prn; stimulate

Reassessment and Ventilation Support

60 sec	HR >100; labored breathing Persistent cyanosis	→	Clear airway, SpO_2, consider CPAP; ongoing assessment
	HR <100 (but >60) or gasping or apnea	→	PPV 40–60 bpm, SpO_2 monitoring

Continued

90 sec	HR <100 (but >60) despite PPV	→	Take ventilation corrective steps; ongoing assessment
	HR <60 despite ventilation corrective steps	→	CPR 120 events*/min; PPV; consider ETT
	If HR remains <60 despite PPV and adequate chest compressions	→	IV epinephrine**; continue CPR; PPV; ETT if no chest rise

*Coordinate 90 compressions and 30 bpm in a 3:1 ratio.

**Epinephrine (1:10,000): 0.01–0.03 mg/kg (0.1–0.3 mL/kg). Give rapidly UVC (preferred), IV or IO (ET route: 0.05–0.1 mg/kg).

Newborn—Emergency Drug Reference

Note: Follow all drugs with 0.5–1.0 mL normal saline flush.

During Resuscitation Efforts

- **Epinephrine (1:10,000):** [bradycardia, asystole] 0.01–0.03 mg/kg IV, IO, umbilicus (consider 0.05–0.1 mg/kg for ET route).
- **NS or LR:** 10 mL/kg IV, IO, or umbilicus over 5–10 min.

Special Consideration—After Restoring Vital Signs

- **Dextrose 10% (D10):** [hypoglycemia] 0.2 g/kg IV only.
- **Sodium Bicarbonate 4.2%:** [confirmed acidosis] 1–2 mEq/kg slow IV, IO (dilute 8.4% with equal amount of NS for 4.2%); use only if newborn is effectively ventilated.

Newborn—Equipment Size and Insertion Depth

Gestational age (wk)	<28	28–34	34–38	>38
Weight (kg)	<1	1–2	2–3	>3
Tracheal tube (mm)	2.5	3.0	3.5	3.5–4.0
ET insertion depth (cm from upper lip)	6–7	7–8	8–9	9–10
Laryngoscope (straight)	0	0	0–1	1
Suction catheter (ET) (French)	5–6	6–8	8	8–10

Newborn: Initial Care and Assessment

NCLEX ABCs, Temperature, and Vital Signs

- Newborn should be pink (for dark skinned Pts, assess oral mucosa, conjunctivae, palms, soles of feet, etc.) and have a loud, vigorous cry.
- Suction nose and mouth to clear excess secretions or mucus.
- Stimulate breathing with vigorous rubbing and drying.
- NCLEX Dry newborn and maintain warmth.
- Assess and document temp and vital signs.

	RR (breaths/min)	HR (bpm)	SBP (mm Hg)	Temp (°C)
Preterm	50–70	140–180	40–60	36.8–37.5
Newborn	30–60	120–160	60–90	36.8–37.5

APGAR Score

- Document APGAR score at 1 and 5 min after delivery.
- **Note:** Some hospitals also require a 10-min APGAR score.

Component	**Interval**	
Appearance (color)	**1 min**	**5 min**
Pink torso and extremities 2		
Pink torso, blue extremities 1		
Blue all over 0		
Pulse (HR)	**1 min**	**5 min**
>100 2		
<100 1		
Absent 0		
Grimace (irritability/reflexes)	**1 min**	**5 min**
Vigorous cry 2		
Limited cry 1		
No response to stimulus 0		

Continued

Component	Interval	
Activity (muscle tone)	**1 min**	**5 min**
Actively moving . . . . 2 Limited movement . . . . 1 Flaccid 0		
Respiratory Effort	**1 min**	**5 min**
Strong, loud cry . . . . 2 Hypoventilation, irregular . . . . 1 Absent 0		
Totals*	**1 min**	**5 min**

*Normal: 8–10; moderate depression: 4–6; aggressive resuscitation: 0–3.

NCLEX Identification and Infant Safety

- Place ID bands on newborn and mother immediately after delivery.
- Record newborn's footprints in chart.
- Always transport newborn in a bassinette.
- Only staff with proper identification may take newborn from mother.

Measurements

- **Weight**: Normal is 6–10 lb.
- **Length**: Normal is 18–22 in.
- **Head circumference**: Normal is 13–14 in. (33–35 cm).
- **Chest circumference**: Normal is 12–13 in. (30–33 cm).

Physical Assessment

◎ Note: Perform regular, head-to-toe assessment, similar to an adult, but note the following areas specific to newborn assessment.

- **Appearance**: Newborn should be pink (for dark skinned Pts, assess oral mucosa, conjunctivae, palms, soles of feet, etc.), have a loud, vigorous cry, and be well flexed with full range of motion and spontaneous movements.
- **Fontanels**: Anterior is diamond shaped, ~4 cm at widest point (closes at 12–18 mo); posterior is triangular, ≤1 cm at widest point (closes at 2–3 mo).
- **Molding**: Skull may be oddly shaped with overlapping cranial bones.

- **Mouth:** Inspect mouth for cleft lip and/or cleft palate.
- **Heart murmur:** Soft murmur is considered normal in first few days.
- **Breathing:** Abdominal breathing is normal in newborns.
- **Umbilical cord:** It should have one vein and two arteries. It is clamped, may or may not be pulsating, and shows no sign of bleeding.
- **Extremities:** Legs and arms are equal in length to each other, and all fingers and toes are present.
- **Male genitalia:** Testes are palpable in scrotum or inguinal canal.
- **Female genitalia:** Large labia minora and vaginal discharge of blood or mucus are considered normal.

Routine Infant Reflexes

Reflex	Stimulation	Response	Age
Babinski's	Stroked sole of foot.	Toes open/fanning upward.	0–12 mo
Galant's	Stroked along spine.	Back arching toward stimulus.	0–6 mo
Grasping (palmar)	Object placed in palm.	Grasping objects.	0–6 mo
Moro's (startle)	Loud noise.	Rapid outward extension of arms followed by a return to midline.	0–2 mo
Parachute	Suspended in prone position (as if falling).	Extension of extremities.	8 mo–adult
Plantar	Stroked ball of foot.	Toes curling downward.	0–12 mo
Rooting	Stroked cheek.	Turning toward stimulus.	0–4 mo

Routine Newborn Medication and Labs

- NCLEX **Eyes:** Antibiotic ointment is administered per hospital policy.
- NCLEX **Vitamin K injection:** This is given to prevent hemorrhage.
- PKU (phenylketonuria): Test results should be obtained 24 hr after feeding begins. Normal serum blood level is <4 mg/dL. Sample is obtained from heel stick.

mother formed harmful antibodies against her fetus's RBCs and transferred them to the fetus via placenta. A heel stick sample is used.

- NCLEX **Immunizations:** Physician may order first hepatitis B vaccine (Hep-B) to be given soon after birth, before discharge.

Mother: Postpartum Care and Assessment

- Monitor for signs of postpartum hemorrhage and shock.
- If pre-eclamptic, assess BP every hour.
- NCLEX Slight fever (100.4°F) is considered normal for first 24 hr postpartum; temp >101.4°F indicates infection.
- Urinary retention is likely postpartum; encourage fluids and monitor I&O for first 12 hr.
- Encourage early ambulation; instruct Pt to change position slowly, because postural hypotension is common postpartum.

Abdomen and Uterus

- The uterus should be firm, about the size of a grapefruit, centrally located, and at the level of the umbilicus immediately postpartum.
- Deviation to the right may indicate distended bladder.
- If postvoid uterus is still boggy, massage top of fundus with fingers held together and reassess every 15 min.
- Assess for bladder fullness (full bladder may inhibit uterine contractions and cause uterine bleeding). Have mother void if bladder is full.
- Mother and/or partner may be instructed to massage fundus.
- Auscultate bowel sounds and inquire daily about BMs.
- Constipation is common from anesthesia and analgesics as is fear of perineal pain.
- Increased fiber and fluid intake, along with early and routine ambulation, will help reduce constipation.

Involution of the Uterus

- Immediately after delivery and within a few hours, the uterus should rise to the level of the umbilicus and remain there for the first 24 hr.
- After this, it descends ~1 cm/day into the pelvic cavity.
- By day 10, it should no longer be palpable in the abdominal cavity.

Breasts and Breastfeeding

- Colostrum appears within 12 hr, and milk appears in ~72 hr postpartum. Breasts become engorged by postpartum day 3 or 4 and should subside spontaneously within 24 to 36 hr.
- Assess breasts for infection and assess nipples for irritation.
- Encourage use of bra between feedings.

Complications

- **Pain:** Assess for mastitis, abscess, milk plug, thrush, etc. Proper positioning of infant (football carry) minimizes soreness. Breast shields prevent clothing from rubbing on nipples.
- NCLEX **Engorgement:** Apply moist heat for 5 min before breastfeeding. Use ice compress after each feeding to reduce swelling and discomfort. Avoid bottles and pacifiers while breasts are engorged because it may cause nipple confusion or preference.
- NCLEX **Mastitis:** Encourage rest and continuation of feeding or pumping. Administer prescribed antibiotics. Note: Breast milk is not infected and will not harm infant.

NCLEX Emotional Status

- Explain to mother and her family that her emotions may shift from high to low and that these changes are considered a normal result of tremendous hormonal changes postpartum.
- Assess parent–infant bonding and family support system.

Lower Extremities

- NCLEX **Thrombophlebitis:** Unilateral swelling, decreased pulses, redness, heat, tenderness, and positive Homans' sign (calf pain or tenderness on dorsiflexion of foot). Leg exercises and early ambulation help minimize occurrence of venous stasis and clot formation.

Perineum

- NCLEX **Episiotomy:** Assess for swelling, bleeding, and infection.
- **Hemorrhoids:** Encourage sitz baths to help reduce discomfort.
- NCLEX **Lochia:** Assess amount, character, and color. Explain stages and duration of lochial discharge, and instruct Pt to report any odor.
  - **Lochia rubra:** Seen 1–3 days postpartum, this is mostly blood and clots.
  - **Lochia serosa:** Seen 4–10 days postpartum, this is serosanguineous.
  - **Lochia alba:** Seen 11–21 days postpartum, this is creamy white and scant

Pediatric Quick Reference (Vitals—Equipment—Electricity)

ge	Term	2 mo	4 mo	6 mo	1 yr	3 yr	6 yr	8 yr	10 yr	11 yr	12 yr
ength (in.)	18–20	20–22	22–24	24–27	27–30	30–33	33–38	38–43	43–48	48–52	>52
Veight (lb)	7	9	11	13–15	18–20	22–24	26–31	33–40	42–48	53–62	66–79
Veight (kg)	3	4	5	6–7	8–9	10–11	12–14	15–18	19–22	24–28	30–36
BP (lower limit)	>60	>60	>60	>60	>70	>76	>82	>86	>90	>90	>90
BP (critical)	<50	<50	<50	<50	<50	<50	<60	<60	<70	<70	<70
eart Rate	85–205	85–205	99–190	99–190	99–190	60–140	60–140	60–140	60–100	60–100	60–100
espiratory Rate	30–60	30–60	30–60	30–60	24–40	22–34	18–30	18–30	18–30	18–30	12–16
aryngoscope Blade*	*straight blade only						*straight or curved				
	1	1	1	1	1	1	2	2	2	2	3
TT (mm, cuffed)	3.0	3.0	3.0	3.0	3.0	4.0	4.5	5.0	5.5	6.0	6.0
TT (mm, uncuffed)	3.5	3.5	3.5	3.5	4.0	5.0	5.5	6.0	6.5	7.0	7.0
TT Insertion Depth cm at gums/teeth)	9–10.5	9–10.5	9–10.5	9–10.5	9–12	12–15	14–17	15–18	17–20	18–21	18–21
efibrillate: 2 J/kg **efibrillate:** 4 J/kg	6 12	8 16	10 20	13 26	17 34	20 40	26 52	33 66	40 80	53 106	66 132
ardiovert: 0.5–1 J/kg **ardiovert:** 2 J/kg	3 6	4 8	5 10	7 13	9 17	10 20	13 26	17 33	20 40	27 53	33 66

Advanced Pediatric Life Support (PALS 2010)

Bradycardia (HR <60 bpm)—Poor Perfusion

Asymptomatic

- Observe and support ABCs as needed.

Symptomatic—Severe Cardiopulmonary Compromise

- Maintain patent airway. Assist breathing as needed.
- Administer oxygen; attach monitor/defibrillator; obtain IV/IO access.
- **CPR**: 2 minutes; begin chest compressions if HR <60/min with poor perfusion despite adequate ventilation and oxygenation; ratio: 30:2 (15:2 if 2 rescuers).
- **Epinephrine:** IV or IO [1:10,000] 0.01 mg/kg (0.1 mL/kg) every 3–5 min; ET [1:1000] 0.1 mg/kg (0.1 mL/kg) every 3–5 min.
- For increased vagal tone or primary AV block, give **atropine:** 0.02 mg/kg IV or OI, may repeat one time. Minimum single dose is 0.1 mg. Maximum total dose is 1 mg.
- **Consider cardiac pacing**: Same as adults, but use pediatric pads, placed anterior to posterior, set rate to 100 bpm.

Tachycardia—Poor Perfusion

Narrow—Complex (≤0.09 sec)

Sinus Tachycardia	
History	Known cause
HR	Infant: <220; child <180
P waves	Normal
PRI	Constant
R—R interval	Variable

- Search for and treat underlying cause.

SVT—Consider Vagal Maneuvers	
History	Vague, sudden onset
HR	Infant: ≥220; child ≥180
HR	Not variable with activity
P waves	Absent, abnormal

- **If IV/IO access:** Adenosine: 0.1 mg/kg (max 1st dose 6 mg) rapid IV push; may give 2nd dose at 0.2 mg/kg (max 2nd dose 12 mg).
- **No IV/IO access:** Synchronized cardioversion: 0.5–1 J/kg; may repeat at 2 J/kg.

Wide—Complex (>0.09 sec)

Probable VT—with cardiopulmonary compromise (e.g., hypotension, AMS, signs of shock)

- Synchronized cardioversion: 0.5–1 J/kg; may repeat at 2 J/kg.

Probable VT—without compromise

- Consider adenosine if rhythm is regular and QRS monomorphic—obtain expert consultation.
- **Antiarrhythmic (one only):** Do not routinely administer amiodarone/procainamide together.
- **Amiodarone:** 5 mg/kg IV/IO over 20–60 min.
- **Procainamide:** 15 mg/kg IV/IO over 30–60 min.
- Torsade/hypomagnesemia: **Magnesium:** 25–50 mg/kg over 10–20 min (max 2 g).

Cardiac Arrest

Asystole—Pulseless Electrical Activity

- **CPR:** 2 min—obtain IV/IO access.
- **Epinephrine:** IV/IO [1:10,000] 0.01 mg/kg (0.1 mL/kg) every 3–5 min; ET [1:1000] 0.1 mg/kg (0.1 mL/kg) every 3–5 min—consider advanced airway.
- **Continue CPR**—rhythm check every 2 min; epinephrine every 3–5 min.
- Search for and manage reversible causes.

V-Fib/Pulseless VT

- **Shock:** Initially 2 J/kg; all subsequent shocks at 4 J/kg (max 10 J/kg).
- **CPR:** 2 min—obtain IV/IO access; reassess rhythm.
- **Shock:** 4 J/kg (max 10 J/kg)—resume CPR.

- **CPR**: 2 min—epinephrine: IV/IO [1:10,000] 0.01 mg/kg (0.1 mL/kg) every 3–5 min; ET [1:1000] 0.1 mg/kg (0.1 mL/kg) every 3–5 min—consider advanced airway; reassess rhythm.
- **Shock**: 4 J/kg (max 10 J/kg)—resume CPR.
- **CPR**: 2 min—amiodarone: 5 mg/kg IV/IO bolus (without interrupting CPR); treat reversible causes. Note: If amiodarone is unavailable, give lidocaine: 1 mg/kg IV/IO (2–3 mg/kg ET). For **Torsade de Pointes,** give magnesium: 25–50 mg/kg IV/IO (max 2 g).

Pediatric Formulas (>1 year)

Systolic BP*	(2 × age in yr) + 90
Diastolic BP*	Approximately 2/3 of the SBP
Weight (kg)	(2 × age in yr) + 8
ET Tube Size (uncuffed)	(Age in yr/4) + 4
ET Tube Size (cuffed)	(Age in yr/4) + 3
ET Tube Depth of Insertion	3 × ET size
Suction Catheter (French)	2 × ET size
Fluid Bolus	10–20 mL/kg

*Capillary refill is acceptable for children younger than 3 years.

Assessment of the Pediatric Patient

- Begin by obtaining history from child's parent(s) and work toward physical assessment. Use this time to establish trust.
- Have parent hold child as much as possible during assessment.
- Approach child at his or her eye level and use first name frequently.
- Use simple language appropriate for child's developmental level.
- Begin assessment with diversion such as toy or game.
- Demonstrate procedures on doll whenever possible.
- Always tell the truth, especially when it comes to painful procedures.
- Perform invasive or uncomfortable assessments at end of assessment.
- Be friendly, but assertive. Do not give child choice when none exists (e.g., "I'm going to look in your mouth" versus "May I look in your mouth?").

Signs and Symptoms by Developmental Stage

- **Infant**: Grimacing; frowning; startled expression; flinching; high-pitched, harsh cry; generalized total body response; possible thrashing of extremities; tremors; increased HR and BP; decreased oxygen saturation.
- **Toddler**: Guarding, possible touching or rubbing of area, generalized restlessness, loud cry, increased HR and BP, possible verbalizing such as "owie" or "boo-boo."
- **Preschooler**: Possible perception of pain as punishment or denial of pain to avoid treatment, possible ability to describe location and intensity, possible crying, kicking, or withdrawal.
- **School-aged child**: Fear of bodily harm and mutilation, awareness of death, ability to describe pain, possible stiff body posture, possible withdrawal or attempt to delay procedures.
- **Adolescent**: Pain perception at physical, emotional, and mental levels, ability to describe pain, possible increased muscle tension, possible withdrawal, and possible decreased motor activity.

Nonpharmacological Interventions for Pain

- **Distraction**: Music, TV, games, dolls, stuffed animals, art, among others.
- **Minimize environmental stimuli**: Noises, bright lights, among others.
- **Provide comfort**: Positioning, rest, and relaxation.
- **Cutaneous stimulation**: Massage or heat or cold therapy.
- **Guided imagery**: Guiding of child to either a make-believe place or someplace visited in the past (e.g., Disneyland).

Be Alert! Respiratory Distress in Pediatrics

Clinical Signs

- Anxiety and/or restlessness.
- Increased respiratory rate and HR.
- Cyanosis (circumoral, mucous membranes, nailbeds).
- Cool, moist skin.
- Nasal flaring, chest wall and sternal retractions.

Abnormal Respiratory Sounds

- **Grunting**: Response to pain; also associated with pulmonary edema.
- **Stridor**: Upper airway involvement; associated with epiglottitis or laryngospasm.
- **Wheezing**: Lower airway involvement; associated with asthma (bilateral) or aspiration of foreign body if unilateral.

Developmental Milestones

Age	Milestone
1 mo	Cries to communicate, has reflex activity, makes eye contact.
2 mo	Coos, smiles, frowns, tracks objects, lifts head.
3 mo	Turns from back to side, sits with support.
4 mo	Turns from back to abdomen, lifts head, bears weight on forearms, can hold head erect, places everything in mouth, grasps with both hands, laughs.
5–6 mo	Turns onto back, uses hands independently, plays with toes, puts feet into mouth, sits alone while leaning forward on hands, holds bottle, extends arms to be picked up, shows stranger anxiety.
7–8 mo	Begins to crawl, bears weight on feet when supported, pulls to a standing position, sits alone without support, has increased fear of strangers, walks alongside furniture, has well-developed crawl.
9–10 mo	May begin to walk and climb; has one- to two-word vocabulary; understands "No!"; shakes head to indicate "No!"; follows simple directions.
12 mo	Walks alone or with assistance, falls frequently while walking, points with one finger.
15–18 mo	Walks independently, throws overhand, pulls/pushes toys, builds with blocks, runs clumsily, jumps in place on both feet, has 8- to 10-word vocabulary.
2 yr	Runs well, climbs stairs, is bladder and bowel (potty) trained, names objects, uses two- or three-word phrases.
3–4 yr	Rides tricycle, turns doorknobs, dresses self, uses short sentences, hops on one foot, can catch a ball.
6–12 yr	Is physically coordinated, uses complete sentences, has extensive vocabulary, swims, skates, rides bicycle, uses complex sentences, reads, forms social groups.

Health History

Chief Complaint

- What prompted parents to bring child to hospital?

- P: Precipitating or palliative factors.
- Q: Quality/quantity; describe symptom(s): Are ADLs affected?
- R: Radiation/region/related symptoms.
- S: Severity: Is symptom mild, moderate, or severe?
- T: Timing; frequency and duration.

Current Intake and Output

- Document last oral intake. Has child been drinking and eating normally?
- Assess for malnutrition and dehydration.
- Does urine and stool output seem normal?

Allergies

- Has child ever had allergic reaction to food, meds, and so on?
- What types of reactions occur with known allergies?

Medications

- Is child currently taking any medications? (Include OTC and prescription medications and herbal remedies.)
- What was time and dose of last medication taken?

Past Medical History

- Prior illnesses and injuries.
- Past or recent hospitalizations and surgical procedures.
- Overall health status since birth.

Events Surrounding Illness or Injury

- History and onset of current illness.
- History and mechanism of injury.

Immunization History

- Are immunizations up to date?
- Has child ever been diagnosed with a communicable disease?
- Has child been recently exposed to a communicable disease?

Injections (IM) for Pediatric Patients

	Muscle*	Needle Size	Max Volume
Infant	NCLEX Vastus lateralis	5/8–7/8″	1 mL
Toddler	Ventrogluteal or vastus lateralis	5/8–1″	1 mL
Older Child	Ventrogluteal or deltoid	5/8–1″	1 mL

*Dorsogluteal site is contraindicated in infants and children.

Recurrent Childhood Illnesses

Chickenpox (Varicella)

- **S/S**: Red pimple-like spots, starting on trunk and spreading to body; pimples progress to red teardrop blisters and eventually break open and scab over.
- Supportive care, standard precautions.

Croup

- **S/S**: Gradual onset, usually at night (fall and winter), with low-grade fever, harsh, "barking seal" cough, hoarse voice; Pt may have sore throat or chest discomfort from coughing.
- Avoid examining airway. Cool, nebulized mist, racemic epinephrine, IV fluids, and steroids may be ordered.

Epiglottitis

- **S/S**: Rapid onset, high-grade fever, inspiratory stridor, muffled voice, difficulty breathing, upright, leaning forward, difficult and painful swallowing, excessive drooling.
- Do not examine airway! Give oxygen, minimize agitation, and be prepared to ventilate with bag valve mask or assist with intubation if airway obstructs.

Gastroenteritis

- **S/S**: Abdominal cramping, bloating, diarrhea (may be bloody and contain mucus), nausea and vomiting, fever and dehydration.
- Supportive care, IV fluids and antiemetics as ordered.

Measles (Rubella)

- **S/S**: Koplik's spots (small, red spots with bluish white centers), progressing to red, blotchy rash along hairline and behind ears, and rapidly spreading to chest and back and then thighs and feet.
- Supportive care, strict standard and airborne precautions.

Meningitis

- **S/S**: Stiff neck, headache, high fever, vomiting, confusion, drowsiness, lethargy, seizures, rash near axilla, hands, and feet, small hemorrhages under skin (petechiae).
- Supportive care, strict standard precautions.

Respiratory Syncytial Virus (RSV)

- **S/S child <3 yr old:** High fever, severe cough, tachypnea, expiratory wheezes, orthopnea.
- **S/S child >3 yr old:** Congestion, runny nose, cough, sore throat, low-grade

Head-Tilt—Chin-Lift: Adult/Child

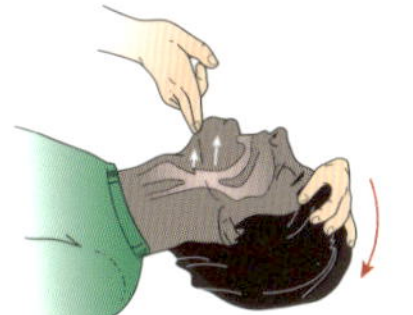

Jaw-Thrust Maneuver
(Known or Suspected Trauma)

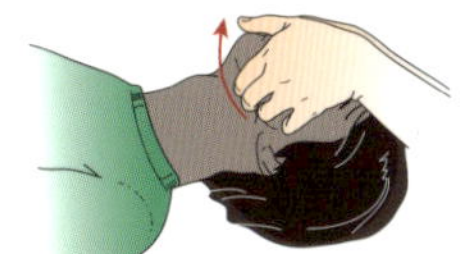

Pulse Check: Adult/Child
(Carotid)

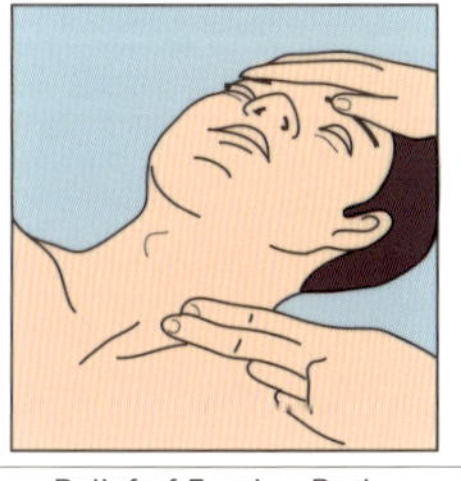

Hand Placement: Adult/Child
(Lower Half of Sternum [Use Heel of One Hand for Child])

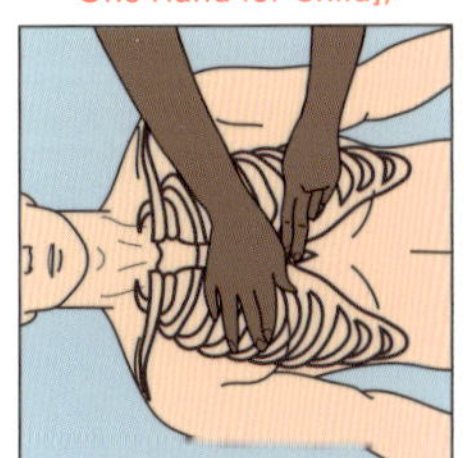

Relief of Foreign Body:
Conscious Adult/Child
(Use Chest Thrusts for Pregnant or Obese Pts)

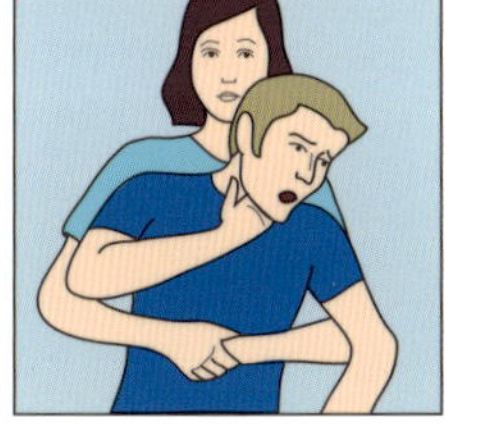

Relief of Foreign Body:
Unresponsive Adult/Child
(Same as for CPR)

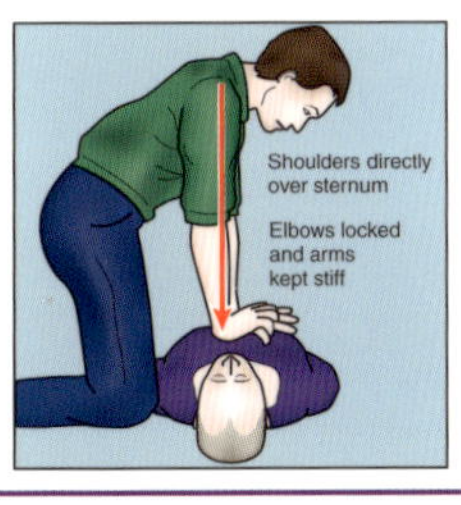

Cardiopulmonary Resuscitation (CPR) Maneuvers

Head-Tilt—Chin-Lift: Infants
(Do Not Hyperextend Neck)

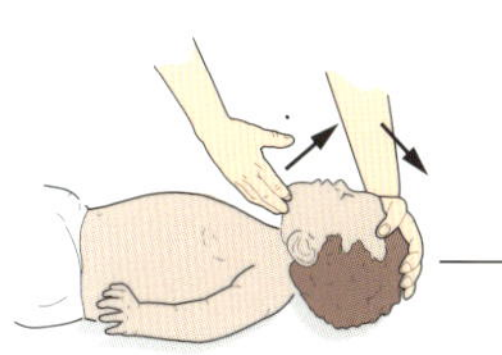

Pulse Check: Infants
(Brachial)

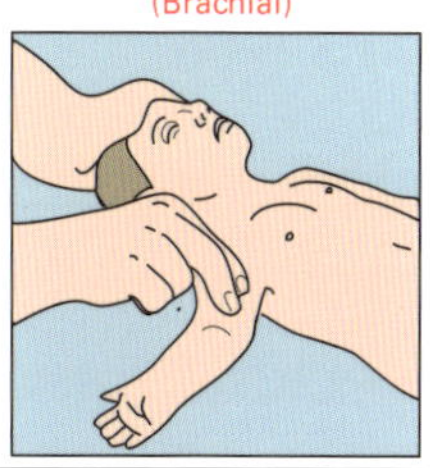

Back Blows and Chest Thrusts: Infants
(Always Support Infant's Head and Neck)

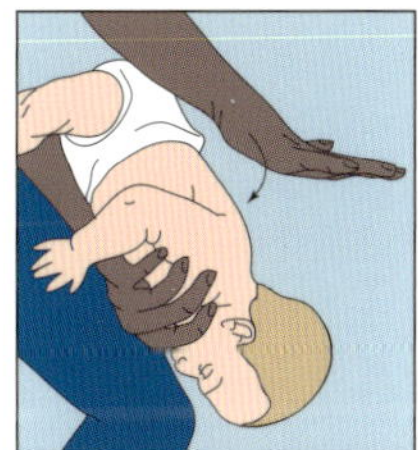

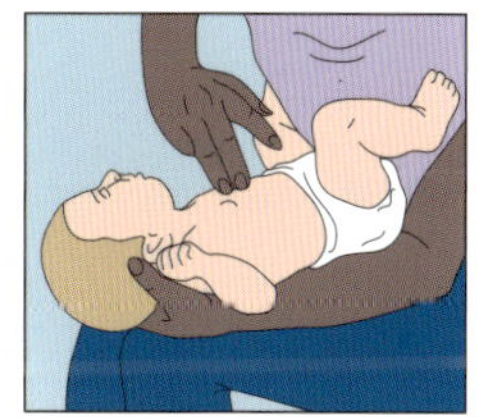

One Rescuer
(One Finger Width Below Nipples)

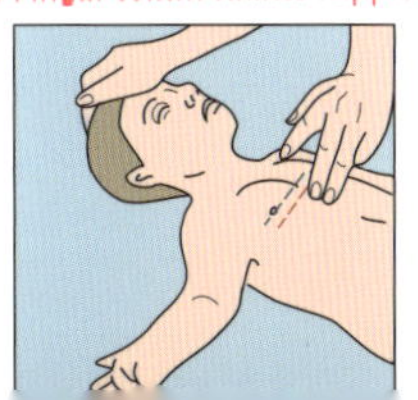

Two Rescuers
(Both Thumbs, Hands Encircling Chest)

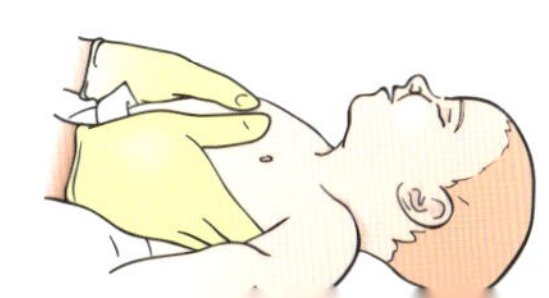

	Adult*	Child*	Infant*
Pulse Check (HCP Only)	Carotid.	Carotid or femoral.	Brachial (NB: umbilicus).
Compression Landmarks	Between nipples, lower half of sternum—child: one hand; adult: two hands, one atop the other.		Just below the nipple line: use two fingers.
Compression Rate	100/min.	100/min.	100/min (NB: 120/min).
Compression Depth	≥2 in.	~⅓ AP diameter.	~⅓ AP diameter.
Airway (All Ages)	Head-tilt—chin-lift; jaw-thrust used for suspected trauma (HCP only).		
Compression-to-Ventilation Ratio	30:2 (1 or 2 rescuers) 1 sec/breath.	30:2 (15:2 if 2 rescuers) 1 sec/breath.	30:2 (15:2 if 2 rescuers) NB: 3:1 (1 or 2 rescuers).
Ventilations With Advanced Airway	1 breath every 6–8 sec; asynchronous with chest compressions, visible chest rise, 1 sec/breath.		
Ventilations Only (Pulse, but No Breathing)	1 every 5–6 sec.	1 every 3–5 sec.	1 every 3–5 sec (NB: 40–60/min).
Ventilations if Untrained or Not Proficient	Compressions only! 100/min.	Compressions only! 100/min.	Compressions only! 100/min (NB: 120/min).
Defibrillation	Attach and use AED/defibrillator as soon as available.		

Ensure high-quality CPR: Allow complete recoil of compressions; minimize interruptions; rotate compressors every 2 min; note visible chest rise with ventilations; allow exhalation between breaths.

*Adult: Adolescent (puberty) and older; Child: 1 yr to adolescent; Infant: <1 yr; Newborn (NB): Birth to 1 mo.

AP: Anteroposterior; HCP: Health-care provider.

NCLEX ACLS—Pulseless Arrest (p. 131); Unstable Arrhythmias (pp. 143–144); Stable Arrhythmias (pp. 144–145)

NCLEX Cardiopulmonary Resuscitation: 2010 Guidelines

Recognition and Activation of EMS

- Victim is unresponsive and not breathing or not breathing normally.
- Activate emergency response system.

Pulse Check: No More Than 10 sec

- **Absent**: 30 compressions and 2 breaths (15:2 if 2 rescuers for child/infant).
- **Present, but not breathing**: Begin rescue breathing—1 breath every 5–6 sec (1 breath every 3–5 sec for child/infant).

CPR (C-A-B)

- **Compressions**: 30 compressions (15, if 2 rescuers for child/infant).
- **Airway**: Open airway with head-tilt—chin-lift or jaw-thrust.
- **Breathing**: Not breathing—give 2 breaths; breathing—recovery position.

Defibrillation—Use AED/Defibrillator as Soon as Available

- **Adult**: Do not use pediatric pads (must be >8 yr or >80 lb).
- **Child/infant**: May use adult pads if pediatric pads are unavailable.
- Recheck pulse after every 2 min of CPR.

NCLEX Choking: 2010 Guidelines

Conscious Victim

- If Pt able to cough effectively, encourage coughing.
- If unable to talk or cough effectively:
  - **Adult or child**: Perform abdominal thrusts (chest thrusts if pregnant or obese) until obstruction is relieved or victim becomes unresponsive.
  - **Infant**: Alternate five back blows and five chest thrusts until obstruction is relieved or victim becomes unresponsive.

Victim Becomes Unresponsive

- Send someone to activate EMS system.
- Lay victim supine and begin CPR (no pulse check).
- Look inside mouth while opening airway—remove obstruction if visible.
- Continue CPR for 5 cycles or 2 min. If you are alone, activate EMS and then resume CPR.
- **Repeat**: Inspect mouth, remove obstruction if seen, give 2 rescue breaths

NCLEX Advanced directives and DNR orders are legal documents that indicate whether a Pt wishes to be resuscitated (and to what extent) in the event of respiratory or cardiac arrest. If any doubt exists about the interpretation or whereabouts of a Pt's advanced directives, then a code must be called and resuscitative efforts initiated.

Clinical Presentation

- Pt who is unresponsive with no detectible respirations or pulse.
- Pt in respiratory arrest (or pre-arrest).
- Pt who has become critically unstable hemodynamically.

Before Arrival of Code Team

- Stay calm! Call out for STAT help or press bedside code button if available. **Note:** Always include floor, unit, and room number.
- Clear immediate Pt area of any obstacles (e.g., tables, chairs).
- Instruct visitors to wait outside the room.
- Begin resuscitation (CPR) while waiting for code team.

After Code Team Has Arrived

- Assist code team resuscitation efforts including compressions, ventilations, medications, defibrillation, or documentation.
- Notify physician or physician on-call and request chaplain to notify and communicate with Pt's family.

Documentation

- All code team members must sign code record.
- Record all times and interventions, and attach ECG strips to code record in chronological order. Clinical tip: Record times and interventions (e.g., drugs, shocks) directly onto ECG strips for easier recall after the code.
- Document a brief summary with outcome in Pt's chart.
- Attach code record to Pt's chart after completed.

Defibrillation and Pacing

Automatic External Defibrillator (AED)

- Turn on AED and follow voice prompts.
- Without interrupting CPR, attach appropriate-sized pads (refer to package insert), and plug pad cable into AED unit if needed.
- Press "Analyze" button (may not be necessary with some models) and wait for instructions.
- If instructed to shock, announce, "Shock indicated, stand clear," and ensure no one is contacting Pt.
- Depress the shock button if prompted.
- Immediately resume CPR and await instruction.

◎ Do not contact Pt while AED is analyzing rhythm.

◎ Do not place electrode over ICD or transdermal medication patch. Remove patch if time permits.

Electrode Size

◎ Do not use pediatric electrodes on adult Pts.

◎ For pediatric and infant Pts, pediatric electrodes with a pediatric attenuator are preferred, but if neither is available, adult electrodes are acceptable.

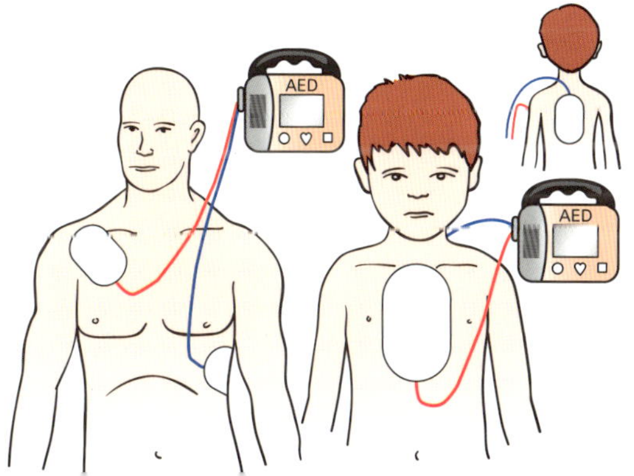

- **Power:** Turn unit on and verify all cables are connected.
- **Lead select:** Turn "lead select" to "paddles" or "defibrillator."
- **Select energy level:** Biphasic: 120–200 J; monophasic: 360.
- Apply conductive medium to paddles, or apply gel pads to Pt's chest.
- **Paddle Placement*:** Sternum (upper right sternal border) and cardiac apex (lower, left-lateral chest). If using hands-free defibrillation pads, follow manufacturer's guidelines (similar to AED—see earlier diagram).
- **Verify rhythm:** Confirm V-Fib or pulseless VT.
- **Charge defibrillator:** Say, "Charging, stand clear!"
- **Clear:** Say, "I'm going to shock on three. One, I'm clear, two, you're clear, three, everybody's clear."
- **Defibrillate:** Biphasic: 120–200 J; monophasic: 360 J.
- **CPR:** Immediately resume CPR for five cycles (about 2 min).
- **Reassess rhythm:** Refer to appropriate algorithm.

Synchronized Electrical Cardioversion

Indication

- Symptomatic stable or unstable tachycardia (with pulses).

Contraindication (When to Use Unsynchronized Mode)

- No pulse, severe prearrest shock, or polymorphic VT.

Technique

- Sedate when clinical situation permits.
- Turn on defibrillator, attach ECG electrodes, press "synch" button, and verify that R-waves are sensed by machine.[1]
- It may be necessary to adjust gain until each R-wave has a synch-marker.
- Select energy level based on arrhythmia.

---

*__Handheld Paddles:__ Apply 25 lb of pressure to both paddles, and depress both paddle discharge buttons simultaneously. **Hands-Free Defibrillation Pads:** Do not contact pads! Depending on type of defibrillator, either press "shock" button on defibrillator or depress both paddle discharge buttons (while docked in defibrillator) simultaneously.

[1]If QRS is too wide for machine to identify R-waves, switch to unsynchronized cardioversion (follow steps for manual defibrillation above).

Rhythm	Waveform	Sequence
Monomorphic VT A-fib	Monophasic	100 J, 200 J, 300 J, 360 J
	Biphasic	100–120 J (escalate as needed)
SVT A-flutter	Monophasic	50 J, 100 J, 200 J, 300 J, 360 J
	Biphasic	100–120 J (escalate as needed)
Polymorphic VT	Monophasic	360 J (treat as pulseless VT)
	Biphasic	120–200 J (high-energy shock)

Monomorphic = all QRS are identical; **polymorphic** = QRS differ in shape.

- **Cardiovert**: Follow same steps[2] for defibrillation (see previous page).
- **Assess rhythm**: Refer to appropriate algorithm for treatment.[3]

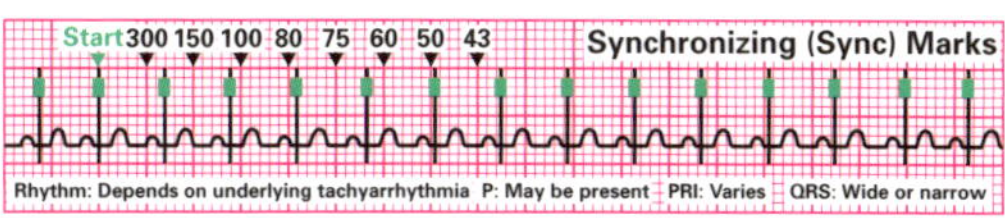

Transcutaneous Pacing

Indications

- Symptomatic 2nd-degree type II or 3rd-degree AV block.
- Symptomatic bradycardia unresponsive to atropine.
- Bradycardia with ventricular escape rhythms.
- May be useful in witnessed rhythm degradation to asystole.
- Overdrive pacing of tachycardia refractory to drug therapy or electrical cardioversion (to be performed by MD only).
- When standby or demand pacing is indicated.

Contraindications

- Severe hypothermia (not recommended for asystole).

Pacing Modes

- Demand (synchronous) mode senses Pt's heart rate and paces only when heart rate falls below predetermined rate.
- Fixed (asynchronous) mode paces at a predetermined rate regardless of Pt's heart rate.

---

[2]Delays are normal. Do not release discharge buttons until shock delivered.
[3]Most defibrillators default back to nonsynchronized mode after each synchronized

- **Power:** Turn on pacemaker and assure cables are connected.
- **Rate:** Set demand rate to 60 bpm and adjust up or down, based on Pt's response, once pacing is initiated.
- **Current:** Output ranges from 0–200 mA.
- **Technique:** Increase mA from minimum setting until consistent capture* is achieved and then increase by 2 mA.

Emergency Medications

Drug	Indication and Dosage
Activated Charcoal	Overdose, Poisoning (see pp. 137–138) **Adults:** 1 g/kg PO, NG. **Peds:** 1 g/kg PO, NG.
Adenosine	SVT (Supraventricular Tachycardia) **Adults/Peds >50 kg:** 6 mg rapid IV, repeat 12 mg × 2. **Peds <50 kg:** 0.1 mg/kg rapid IV, may repeat 0.2 mg/kg. Administration: Record ECG during injection; prepare adenosine and 20 mL NS flush in separate syringes; insert both in same injection port closest to Pt; clamp IV tubing above injection port; inject adenosine as quickly as possible; inject NS flush as quickly as possible; unclamp tubing.
Albuterol	Bronchospasm, Acute Asthma Exacerbation **Adults/Peds >12 yr:** 2.5 mg nebulized every 10 min. **Peds 2–12 yr:** 0.15 mg/kg, repeated as needed.
Amiodarone	Unstable V-Tach **Adults:** 150 mg IV over 10 min. **Peds:** 5 mg/kg over 20–60 min. VF or VT Arrest **Adults:** 300 mg IV, repeat 150 mg. **Peds:** 5 mg/kg IV, max single dose 300 mg.
Aspirin	ACS (Acute Coronary Syndrome) **Adults:** 160–325 mg PO chewable (not enteric coated).

Continued

*Capture is characterized by pacer spikes, a wide QRS, and broad T waves. Avoid using carotid artery to confirm mechanical capture, because muscular jerking (from pacing) can mimic a carotid pulse.

Drug	Indication and Dosage
Atenolol	ACS **Adults:** 5 mg slow IV (over 5 min).
Atropine	Bradycardia **Adults:** 0.5–1 mg IV every 3–5 min, max 3 mg. **Peds:** 0.02 mg/kg IV; may double and repeat once; minimum 0.1 mg, maximum 1 mg.
Dextrose	Hypoglycemia **Adults:** 12.5–25 g slow IV. **Peds:** 0.5–1 g/kg slow IV (D50: 1–2 mL/kg; D25: 2–4 mL/kg; D10: 5–10 mL/kg).
Diazepam	Seizures, Status Epilepticus **Adults:** 5–10 mg slow IV, repeat every 10–15 min, max 30 mg; rectally: 0.2 mg/kg PR. **Peds >1 month:** 0.2 mg/kg slow IV every 2–5 min, max 5 mg; rectally: 0.3 mg/kg PR.
Diltiazem	A-Fib /A-Flutter **Adults:** 15–20 mg slow (2 min) IVP.
Diphenhydramine	Allergic Reaction, Anaphylaxis **Adults:** 25–50 mg IV, IM. **Peds >10 kg:** 1.25 mg/kg.
Dobutamine	Pump Problem, Heart Failure **Adults:** 2–20 mcg/kg/min IV drip. **Peds:** Same as adult dose.
Dopamine	Pump Problem, Heart Failure **Adults:** 2–20 mcg/kg/min IV drip **Peds:** Same as adult dose.
Epinephrine 1:1000 (SC only!)	Bronchospasm **Adults:** 0.3–0.5 mg SC, IM. **Peds:** 0.01 mg/kg (0.01 mL/kg) SC, max 0.5 mg.
Epinephrine 1:10,000	Cardiac Arrest **Adults:** 1 mg IV every 3–5 min. **Peds IV:** 0.01 mg/kg (0.1 mL/kg). **Peds ET:** Use 1:1000 0.1 mg/kg (0.1 mL/kg) ET.
Fentanyl	Pain Management **Adults:** 0.5–1 mcg/kg/dose IV. **Peds:** 1–2 mcg/kg/dose IV. RSI (Rapid Sequence Intubation) **Adults:** 2–10 mcg/kg IV. **Peds:** 0.5–1 mcg/kg IV, max 4 mcg/kg.

Drug	Indication and Dose
Flumazenil	Benzodiazepine Overdose **Adults:** 0.2 mg IV, may repeat 0.3 mg IV in 30 sec, may repeat 0.5 mg IV in 30 sec; max 3 mg. **Peds:** 0.01 mg/kg.
Furosemide	Pulmonary Edema **Adults:** 0.5–1 mg/kg IV (over 1–2 min). **Peds:** 1 mg/kg.
Glucagon	Beta Blocker Overdose, Hypoglycemia **Adults:** 1 mg IV, IM. **Peds <20 kg:** 0.5 mg IV, IM.
Ipratropium 0.02%	Bronchospasm **Adults:** 0.5 mg nebulized with albuterol. **Peds:** 25 mcg/kg nebulized with albuterol.
Isuprel	Bradycardia (Heart Transplant Patients) **Adults:** 2–10 mcg/min IV.
Labetalol	Hypertension, Hypertensive Crisis **Adults:** 10 mg IVP over 1–2 min.
Lidocaine	V-Fib, V-Tach **Adults:** 1–1.5 mg/kg IV, max 3 mg/kg. **Peds:** 1 mg/kg, max 100 mg.
Magnesium	Hypomagnesemia, Torsade de Pointes **Adults:** 1–2 g IV. **Peds:** 20–50 mg/kg (max 2 g) IV over 10–20 min.
Mannitol	Increased ICP (Intracranial Pressure) **Adults:** 0.5–1 g/kg IV over 5–10 min. **Peds:** 0.2–0.5 g/kg over 30–60 min.
Methylprednisolone	Allergic Reaction, Anaphylaxis **Adults:** 1–2 mg/kg IV. **Peds:** Same as adult dose.
Midazolam	Sedative **Adults:** 1–2 mg IV every 2 min. **Peds:** 0.05–0.2 mg/kg.
Morphine	ACS, Pain Management **Adults:** 1–2-mg increments IV. **Peds:** 0.1–0.2 mg/kg.
Naloxone	Narcotic Overdose **Adults:** 0.4–2 mg IV every 2–3 min. **Peds:** 0.1 mg/kg.

Continued

Drug	Indication and Dosage
Nitroglycerin	Ischemic CP, ACS **Adults:** 0.4 mg SL every 3–5 min × 3.
Ondansetron	Nausea **Adults:** 4 mg IV, IM. **Peds: ≤40 kg:** 0.1 mg/kg IV; >40 kg: 4 mg IV, IM.
Procainamide	V-Fib, V-Tach **Adults:** 20–50 mg/min IV, max 17/kg. **Peds:** 15 mg/kg over 30–60 min.
Vasopressin	Asystole, PEA, V-Fib **Adults:** 40 units IV once.

ACS: acute coronary syndrome; **EC**: enteric coated; **PEA**: pulseless electrical activity; **SC**: subcutaneous; **VF, V-Fib**: ventricular fibrillation; **VT, V-Tach**: ventricular tachycardia

Medical Emergencies

Initial Assessment and Intervention for All Pts

Assessment (As Applicable)

- Assess neurological status, level of alertness, level of consciousness.
- Assess airway, respiratory, and circulatory status (ABCs).
- Palpate radial pulse for rate and rhythm and character.
- If Pt monitored, assess ECG and treat arrhythmias per physician order.
- Obtain SAMPLE history.
- Assess baseline VS (HR, RR, BP, SpO_2, temp.).
- Assess pain/symptom characteristics (see OPQRST in ASSESS).

Intervention (As Applicable)

- Establish and maintain ABCs.
- Treat life-threatening emergencies immediately.
- Initiate emergency interventions (e.g., call a code, defibrillation).
- Place Pt in position of comfort and offer reassurance.
- Administer oxygen as indicated/ordered and titrate to SpO_2 >90%.
- Using SBAR format, notify physician of change in Pt status including pertinent assessment findings and any interventions.
- Obtain IV access as ordered and titrate to SBP >90 mm Hg.
- Obtain labs, ECG, and imaging studies as ordered.
- Document assessments, any interventions, and outcome.

Clinical Findings

Neuro: Anxiety, restlessness.
Resp: Increased respiratory rate and/or distress.
CV: Increased heart rate and/or hypotension.
Skin: Fever and/or coolness, pallor, and diaphoresis.
GI/GU: Anorexia; hyperactive, hypoactive, or absent bowel sounds; nausea, vomiting, diarrhea, constipation, GI bleeding.
MS: Abdominal tenderness, distention, rigidity, guarding, flank pain, palpable pulsatile mass, fatigue, malaise.

Collaborative Management

- Inquire about recent bowel habits including laxatives or enemas.
- Inspect abdomen for symmetry and distention.
- Auscultate bowel sounds (hyperactive/hypoactive or absent).
- Palpate all abdominal quadrants for masses, pulsations, tenderness, and rigidity (from area of least tenderness to area of most tenderness).
- Assess NG tube placement and output if present.
- Assess indwelling urinary catheter if present to ensure drainage, and record amount, color, and clarity of urine (consider bladder scan if no catheter).
- Obtain STAT bedside blood glucose level if Pt has diabetes.
- Test emesis/NG drainage and/or stool for occult blood.
- Administer antiemetic and pain medication if ordered.
- Insert NG tube and initiate nasogastric suctioning as ordered.
- Perform bladder scan and/or insert urinary catheter as ordered.

Allergic Reaction: Anaphylaxis

Clinical Findings

Neuro: Anxiety, restlessness.
Resp: Dyspnea, bronchospasm, wheezing, stridor, swelling of tongue or throat, respiratory arrest.
CV: Hypotension, localized or systemic edema, CV collapse.
Skin: Rash, itching, hives, coolness, pallor, cyanosis, diaphoresis.

Collaborative Management

- Remove source of allergic reaction (e.g., IV infusion, latex gloves).
- If Pt is receiving blood transfusion, see Transfusion Reaction (see later).
- Monitor airway, respiratory, and circulatory status closely.

- Assess for edema (specifically facial, lips, tongue, throat).
- Administer or assist with STAT medication as ordered, by severity*:

Severity	Pharmacological Intervention
Mild: Itching, rash or hives only.	**Diphenhydramine**: 25–50 mg IV, IM. **Cimetidine**: 300 mg IV, IM, PO.
Moderate: Above s/s plus swelling of lips or tongue.	**Dexamethasone**: 10 mg IV, IM *or* **Methylprednisolone**: 40–125 mg IV, IM. **Albuterol**: 2.5 mg nebulized in 3 mL NS.
Severe: Above s/s plus dyspnea.	**Epinephrine** (1:1000) 0.3–0.5 mg SC.
Critical: Above s/s plus airway closure, hypotension (anaphylaxis).	**IV fluids**: Goal SBP >90 mm Hg. **Epinephrine** (1:10,000) 0.1–0.25 mg IV. **Dopamine**: Start at 10 mcg/kg/min. **Glucagon**: 1 mg IV over 5 min (if unresponsive to epinephrine or Pt is taking beta blockers).

Altered Mental Status (AMS)

Clinical Findings

Neuro: Confused, lethargic, obtunded, stuporous, or comatose.

Resp: Depressed (likely opioid OD), Cheyne-Stokes breathing (likely CVA), Kussmaul's respirations or fruity odor on breath (likely DKA), apneustic (likely brainstem injury), odor of alcohol (likely intoxication), sweet almond odor (likely cyanide exposure).

CV: Increased BP and decreased HR (likely increased ICP), hypotension (likely sepsis, MI, OD, internal bleeding), dysrhythmias.

Skin: Cool and moist (likely hypoglycemia, vasovagal response, MI, shock), warm and flushed (likely spinal injury, hyperglycemia, sepsis).

GI/GU: Nausea and vomiting, incontinence.

MS: Weakness, fatigue, abnormal flexion or extension, trauma.

Collaborative Management

- Place in lateral-lying position and suction airway as needed.
- Assess pupils and establish baseline GCS score.
- Assess for neurological deficits (e.g., slurred speech, facial droop, or weakness or numbness on one side of the body).
- Obtain STAT bedside blood glucose level.
- Review MAR and labs for causes of AMS.
- Administer or assist with STAT medication as ordered:

Hypoglycemia	Glucose 25 g IV.
Narcotic OD	Naloxone 0.2–2 mg IV.
Benzodiazepine OD	Flumazenil 0.2 mg IV.

Bradycardia (ACLS)

Clinical Findings

Neuro: Dizziness, light-headedness, AMS, syncope.
Resp: SOB.
CV: HR <60 bpm, hypotension, pulmonary congestion.
Skin: Cyanosis, coolness, pallor, diaphoresis.
GI/GU: Nausea and vomiting.
MS: Weakness, lethargy, fatigue, exhaustion.

Collaborative Management

Stable Bradycardia (ACLS 2010)

- Treatment should not be based on HR alone! If Pt is otherwise asymptomatic (e.g., no CP or SOB, stable BP), implement supportive care measures, notify physician STAT, and search for reversible causes.
- **Note:** Common causes of asymptomatic bradycardia include excellent physical conditioning (e.g., athletes) and medication (e.g., beta blockers, digoxin).
- Assess LOC and orientation.
- Lay Pt flat and elevate feet 10°–15° if Pt is feeling dizzy or faint.
- Assess for associated symptoms (CP, respiratory distress, or hypotension).
- Administer STAT medication as ordered—only if symptomatic.

NCLEX Unstable Bradycardia (HR typically <50 bpm): ACLS 2010

If Pt is unstable (CP, decreased BP, SOB, or AMS), call a code/notify physician STAT. Pt requires immediate intervention!

- Identify and treat underlying cause.
- **Atropine:** Give 0.5 mg IV every 3–5 min to a maximum of 3 mg.
- If atropine ineffective:
  - **Pace:** Begin transcutaneous pacing (Do not delay for 2nd-degree type 2 or 3rd-degree AV block.) or
  - **Dopamine:** 2–10 mcg/kg/min or
  - **Epinephrine:** 2–10 mcg/min infusion.
- Expert consultation: Definitive care may require transvenous pacing.

Cardiac Arrest (ACLS)

Call a code/notify HCP STAT. Pt requires immediate intervention!

- CPR: Push hard and fast, minimize interruptions, and avoid hyperventilation.
- Give oxygen, attach monitor/defibrillator, and assess rhythm.

NCLEX Asystole/PEA (ACLS 2010)

- CPR: 2 min. Obtain IV/IO access.
- **Epinephrine:** 1 mg IV/IO every 3–5 min; consider advanced airway. **Vasopressin:** 40 units IV/IO can replace 1st or 2nd dose of epinephrine.
- Continue CPR, with rhythm check every 2 min and epi every 3–5 min.
- Search for and manage reversible causes.

NCLEX V-Fib or Pulseless VT (ACLS 2010)

- **Shock:** Biphasic, 120–200 J; monophasic, 360 J.
- **CPR:** 2 min—obtain IV/IO access—reassess rhythm.
- **Shock:** Biphasic: 120–200 J; monophasic: 360 J.
- **CPR:** 2 min—**Epinephrine:** 1 mg IV/IO every 3–5 min. Consider advanced airway and reassess rhythm. **Vasopressin:** 40 units IV/IO can replace first or second dose of epinephrine.
- **Shock:** Biphasic: 120–200 J; monophasic: 360 J.
- CPR: 2 min—Amiodarone: 300 mg IV/IO. May repeat (if needed) at 150 mg. Treat reversible causes and reassess rhythm. **Note:** If amiodarone is unavailable, give **lidocaine:** 1.0–1.5 mg/kg IV/IO, repeated 0.5–0.75 mg/kg every 5–10 min, maximum 3 doses or 3 mg/kg.
- For torsade de pointes, give **magnesium:** 1–2 g (diluted in 10 mL) IV/IO.

Reversible Causes	
• **H**ypovolemia	• **T**oxins
• **H**ypoxia	• **T**amponade (cardiac)
• **H**ydrogen ion (acidosis)	• **T**ension pneumothorax
• **H**ypokalemia/hyperkalemia	• **T**hrombosis (coronary)
• **H**ypoglycemia	• **T**hrombosis (pulmonary)
• **H**ypothermia	• **T**rauma

Chest Pain

Clinical Findings

Neuro: Anxiety, restlessness, dizziness, light-headedness, syncope, possible sense of impending doom.

MS: Substernal pain, weakness, fatigue, sensation of chest heaviness or chest tightness.

GI/GU: Nausea and vomiting.

Collaborative Management

- Obtain STAT 12-lead ECG and focused symptom analysis.
- Administer or assist with STAT medication as ordered:

Medication	Dose
Nitroglycerin	0.4 mg SL (hold for BP <90 mm Hg)
Aspirin	160–325 mg chewed (not enteric coated)
Morphine	2–4 mg IV (hold for SBP <90 mm Hg)

Diabetic Emergencies

Clinical Findings

	Hypoglycemia	Hyperglycemia
History	Recent insulin shot, missed meal, excessive exercise.	Infection, stress, trauma, insufficient insulin intake.
Onset	Rapid (minutes)	Gradual (days to weeks).
Neuro	Confusion, delirium, coma, seizures.	Irritability, headache (HA), double or blurred vision.
Resp	Normal respiratory pattern.	Deep and rapid (Kussmaul's).
Breath	Normal (no fruity odor).	Fruity (acetone) odor.
CV	Weak, rapid HR, SBP variable.	HR normal to fast, SBP variable.
Skin	Cool, pale, and diaphoretic.	Warm, dry, flushed.
GI/GU	Nausea and vomiting.	Polydipsia, polyuria, nausea and vomiting, abdominal cramps, dehydration.
MS	Weakness, tremor, twitch.	Muscle wasting.
Blood Glucose	<80 mg/dL.	>180 mg/dL.

Collaborative Management

- Obtain finger-stick blood glucose level.
- Administer or assist with STAT medication as ordered:

Presentation	Medication
Hypoglycemia	Dextrose 50%: 25 g IV.
Hyperglycemia	IV fluid, insulin (potassium as indicated).

Dizziness, Vasovagal Response, Syncope

Clinical Findings

Neuro: Dizziness, light-headedness, faintness, anxiety, syncope.
Resp: SOB, hyperventilation.
CV: Hypotension, tachycardia, bradycardia, CP, chest tightness or pressure, palpitations, dysrhythmias.
Skin: Coolness, pallor, diaphoresis.
GI/GU: Nausea and vomiting.
MS: Weakness, fatigue.

Collaborative Management

- Stay with Pt until you can assist to chair or back to bed (if, during assist, Pt has syncopal episode, assist Pt to floor, call for help, then assess ABCs).
- Lay Pt flat and elevate foot of bed 10°–15°.
- If Pt is hyperventilating, encourage slow, deep breathing.
- Assess for neurological deficits (e.g., slurred speech, unequal pupils, facial droop, or weakness or numbness on one side of the body).
- Assess for associated symptoms (CP, respiratory distress, or hypotension).
- Review MAR and labs for causes of dizziness or syncope.
- Obtain STAT bedside blood glucose level.
- Obtain and document orthostatic vital signs (each set, 1 min apart) from supine, sitting, and standing positions – Use extreme caution (Pt may pass out) and extra staff or specialty equipment (e.g., standing platform) as needed based on Pt's presentation and tolerance to test. **Note**: An increase in HR or decrease in SBP by 20 points from baseline is positive for orthostatic hypotension.

Clinical Findings

Neuro: Dizziness, light-headedness, vertigo, faintness, HA, anxiety, AMS, restlessness, visual disturbances, seizures.
Resp: SOB, hyperventilation.
CV: Tachycardia, bradycardia, CP, palpitations, dysrhythmias, dependent edema, symptoms of CHF.
Skin: Coolness and moisture, warmth and flushing, tingling sensation.
GI/GU: Nausea and vomiting.
MS: Weakness, fatigue.

Collaborative Management

- **Note:** If SPB >220 or DPB >140 mm Hg, notify physician STAT.
- Elevate Pt's head of bed to 30°–45°.
- Assess LOC and orientation.
- Palpate pulse for rate and rhythm. If Pt is monitored, assess ECG.
- Assess for neurological deficits such as slurred speech, unequal pupils, facial droop, or weakness or numbness on one side of body and other associated findings (chest pain; respiratory distress; rapid, thready pulse; or AMS).
- Obtain and record BP readings in both arms.
- Administer or assist with antihypertensive medication as ordered.

Hypotension

Clinical Findings

Neuro: Anxiety, restlessness, dizziness, light-headedness, decreased LOC, faintness, syncope.
Resp: SOB, respiratory distress.
CV: SBP <90 mm Hg, or SBP 40 mm Hg below Pt's normal baseline BP, tachycardia, bradycardia, CP, dysrhythmia.
Skin: Coolness, pallor, diaphoresis.
GI/GU: Nausea and vomiting, UO <30 mL/hr.
MS: Weakness, fatigue.

Collaborative Management

- Lay Pt flat, unless contraindicated by respiratory or airway compromise.
- Elevate foot of bed 10°–15°.
- Assess LOC and orientation.
- Assess for and control any bleeding with direct pressure.
- Anticipate and prepare for return to surgery if Pt is postoperative.
- Assess for associated symptoms (CP, respiratory distress, AMS).
- Review medical record (medication, recent labs, and treatments) for possible causes of drop in BP.

Increasing Intracranial Pressure

Clinical Findings

Cushing's Reflex: Hypertension, bradycardia, unequal pupils, irregular respirations, hyperthermia.
Neuro: AMS, HA, sensitivity to light, irritability, double or blurred vision, seizures, hemiparesis, GCS <8, unequal pupils.
Resp: Abnormal respirations, tachypnea (late).
CV: HTN, Bradycardia (late), widening pulse pressure (late).
GI/GU: Nausea and vomiting.
MS: Weakness, decreased motor function, posturing.

Collaborative Management

- Monitor pupils and GCS.
- Controlled hyperventilation decreases $PaCO_2$, thus causing cerebral vasoconstriction and decreased ICP. **Note:** If capnography monitoring is available, goal should be an $EtCO_2$ of 30 mm Hg.
- Keep head elevated to 30°, maintain head in neutral alignment, and avoid flexion or rotation of neck.
- Closely monitor VS and neurological status.

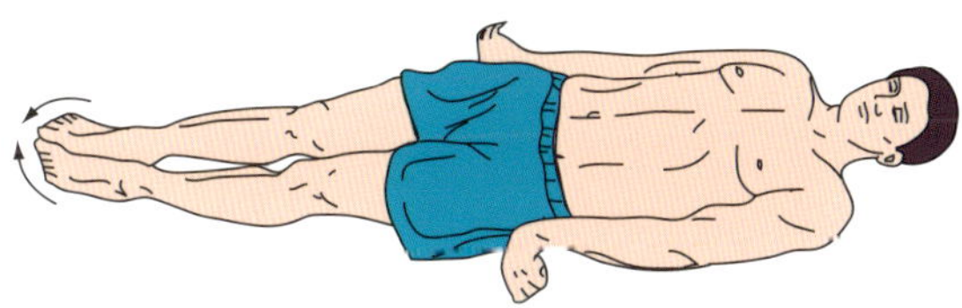

NCLEX Abnormal Extension (decerebrate posturing)

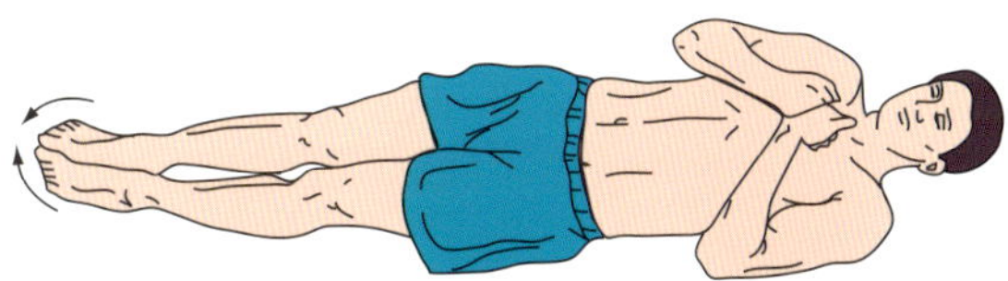

NCLEX Abnormal Flexion (decorticate posturing)

Clinical Findings (Etiological)

Infection: Inflammatory response to microorganisms, especially those that release toxins or invade body tissues.

Fever: Temp >100.4°F (38°C); low-grade: temp. 100.4°–101°F (38.3°C); high-grade: temp. >101°F. **Note**: A patient my not exhibit a fever (normothermic) or may even be hypothermic if septic.

Systemic inflammatory response syndrome (SIRS): Systemic response to any severe clinical insult (e.g., infection, trauma, burns, or pancreatitis) includes two or more of the following:

- Temp >38°C (100.4°F) or <36°C (96.8°F)
- HR >90 bpm
- RR >20 bpm or $PaCO_2$ <32 mm Hg
- WBC count >12,000/mm^3, <4000/mm^3, or presence of >10% immature neutrophils

Sepsis: SIRS is triggered by infection caused when microorganisms (most often bacteria) enter systemic circulation. Symptoms include increased RR (early), fever (may also be hypothermic), chills, increased HR, decreased UO, shivering, skin rash, and warm skin.

Severe sepsis: Sepsis shows evidence of end-organ hypoperfusion (e.g., acute AMS, hypoxia, oliguria [UO <400 mL/day], or lactic acidosis). Complications include impaired blood flow to vital organs and DIC caused by toxins released by microorganisms. The body's own inflammatory response to the release of toxins also contributes to end-organ failure.

Septic shock: Sepsis with life threatening hypotension (SBP <90 mm Hg or a reduction >40 mm Hg from baseline) occurs despite adequate fluid resuscitation or the requirement of vasopressors to maintain BP.

Surgical-site infection (SSI): Localized infection is evidenced by localized redness (or streaking), tenderness, swelling, and warmth as well as fever, purulent or serosanguineous drainage, foul odor, dehiscence, or evisceration.

Collaborative Management

- Monitor temp and vital signs.
- Fever: Offer cold compress to forehead or nape of neck, encourage fluids if not restricted, and administer antipyretic medication as ordered.
- Nausea: Position for comfort, provide emesis basin, offer cold compress to forehead or nape of neck, offer ice chips or small sips of clear liquids if tolerated; otherwise, keep NPO until nausea passes, and administer antinausea medication as ordered.
- Search for potential causes: blood transfusions, surgical and nonsurgical (decubitus ulcers) wounds, surgical drains, indwelling catheters (urinary, peripheral and central IVs).

- Encourage Pt to cough and breathe deeply (incentive spirometer).
- Monitor UO and fluid intake.
- Monitor closely for evidence of end-organ hypoperfusion (e.g., acute AMS, hypoxia, oliguria, and/or lactic acidosis).
- Administer oxygen, IV fluids, and antibiotics as ordered. Pts may also need vasopressors, ventilatory support, blood products, and dialysis.
- Diagnostic tests may include blood cultures (concurrent use of antibiotics can produce false-negative results), WBC, CBC with differential, BUN, creatinine, ABG, platelet count, DIC, and chest x-ray.

Overdose (OD)

Clinical Findings

CNS depressants (opioids, sedatives): Constricted pupils, drowsiness, weakness, coma, respiratory depression, pulmonary edema, apnea, bradycardia, hypotension, hypothermia.

CNS stimulants (cocaine, amphetamines): Dilated pupils, anxiety, agitation, HA, psychosis, tachypnea, tachycardia, dysrhythmias, HTN, CP, diaphoresis, hyperthermia.

Other toxins: Symptoms vary widely depending on type of toxin and can include weakness, fatigue, HA, dizziness, visual disturbances, nausea and vomiting, bradycardia (beta blockers), hypotension (calcium channel blockers), tachycardia (tricyclic antidepressants), abdominal pain, and AMS.

Collaborative Management

- **Protect yourself** from potentially aggressive Pts.
- Anticipate and prepare for respiratory and cardiovascular compromise.
- Position Pt on left side and suction airway as needed (for decreased LOC).
- Definitive treatment requires rapid identification of toxin.
- Administer STAT antidote/reversal as ordered.

Toxin-Specific Treatments

◎ **Caution:** Avoid use of ipecac, because vomiting may complicate or worsen clinical management of OD or poisoning.

Acetaminophen (APAP, Tylenol)

- Supportive care as indicated.
- **Common antidotes:** Activated charcoal and *N*-acetylcysteine.

Aspirin (ASA; Bayer, Excedrin)

- Supportive care as indicated.
- **Common antidotes:** Activated charcoal and sodium bicarbonate 8.4%.

[Tenormin])

- Supportive care as indicated. **Be alert for extreme bradycardia.**
- **Common antidotes:** Activated charcoal and glucagon.

Calcium Channel Blockers (diltiazem [Cardizem], verapamil [Isoptin])

- Supportive care as indicated. **Be alert for hypotension and bradycardia.**
- **Common antidotes:** Activated charcoal and calcium chloride 10%.

CNS Stimulants (cocaine, methamphetamine, speed, crank)

- Protect self and staff, and call for security. Pt may be hostile.
- Minimize sensory stimulation.
- Supportive care as indicated. Treat symptoms of ACS.
- **Common antidotes:** Activated charcoal and midazolam.

Extrapyramidal Symptoms

- Symptoms associated with phenothiazines and tranquilizers.
- Supportive care as indicated.
- **Common antidote:** Diphenhydramine.

Hallucinogens (LSD, PCP, some mushrooms, mescaline, THC)

- Protect self and staff; call for security. Pt may be hostile.
- Minimize sensory stimulation. Provide supportive care as indicated.
- **Common antidote:** Diazepam.

Narcotics/Opioids (heroin, methadone, meperidine [Demerol], oxycodone)

- Protect self and staff; call for security. Pt may be hostile.
- Be prepared to support airway and ventilations as indicated.
- **Common antidote:** Naloxone or nalmefene.

Sedative-Hypnotics (benzodiazepines, flunitrazepam [Rohypnol])

- Be prepared to support airway and ventilations as indicated.
- **Common antidote:** Flumazenil.

Tricyclic Antidepressants (nortriptyline, amitriptyline)

- Watch for tachycardia with widened QRS complex.
- Be prepared to support airway and ventilations as indicated.
- **Common antidote:** Sodium bicarbonate 8.4%

Postoperative Hemorrhage

Clinical Findings

Neuro: Early signs: anxiety, agitation, restlessness, light-headedness; late signs: decreased LOC, confusion.

Resp: SOB, respiratory distress.

CV: Hypotension (late sign), tachycardia, capillary refill >3 sec, diminished peripheral pulses.

Skin: Coolness, pallor, diaphoresis, cyanosis, mottling, ecchymosis.

GI/GU: Rigid, distended abdomen; periumbilical and/or retroperitoneal bruising, nausea, hematemesis, decreased UO, thirst.

MS: Weakness, fatigue.

Incision: Excessive swelling and ecchymosis.

Other: Excessive wound drainage, saturated dressing, melena, excessive blood loss through chest tube or NGT.

Collaborative Management

- Assess for and control external bleeding with direct pressure.
- Get help and notify surgeon STAT.
- Discontinue any thrombolytics or anticoagulants as ordered.
- Reinforce saturated dressing with additional dressing and pressure. (Do not remove saturated dressing.)
- Lay Pt flat unless contraindicated by respiratory or airway compromise.
- Elevate foot of bed 10°–15°.
- Monitor LOC and orientation.
- Obtain and record outputs (surgical drains, urinary catheter).
- Anticipate and prepare for Pt's return to surgery.

Respiratory Distress

Clinical Findings

Neuro: Anxiety, restlessness, confusion, AMS.

Resp: Dyspnea, tachypnea, bradypnea, use of accessory muscles, sternal retractions, wheezing, rales, stridor, coughing.

CV: Tachycardia, dysrhythmias, HTN, pulmonary edema (CHF).

Skin: Cyanosis, coolness, pallor, diaphoresis.

MS: Weakness, lethargy, fatigue, exhaustion, bolt upright or tripod position to facilitate breathing.

- Assess Pt for signs associated with allergic reaction.
- SpO_2 <90% is considered abnormal and may require immediate intervention, but some Pts (e.g., Pts with COPD) can maintain a baseline SpO_2 of 88%–89% and are considered stable. These Pts depend on increased levels of CO_2 to maintain respiratory drive. Use oxygen judiciously when administering supplemental oxygen in presence of COPD, because excessive amounts may decrease Pt's respiratory drive and inevitably cause clinical situation to progress to full respiratory arrest.
- If Pt shows signs of inadequate oxygenation (e.g., AMS, cyanosis) or RR <8 breaths/min, consider inserting nasopharyngeal airway and provide manual ventilations.
- Suction oropharynx and clear secretions as needed.
- If Pt is hyperventilating, encourage slow, deep breathing.
- Obtain focused medical history including recent surgeries and injuries.
- Complete a focused respiratory assessment.
- Administer or assist with STAT medication as ordered.

Seizure

Clinical Findings

Neuro: LOC (blank stare if petit mal seizure).
Resp: Inability to breathe adequately, apnea.
Skin: Cyanosis, coolness and moisture, or warmth and flushing.
MS: Repetitive jerking movements of upper and lower extremities, blinking, deviation of eyes and/or tongue.
GI/GU: Urinary or fecal incontinence.

Seizure Progression

- Aura (before seizure starts): An auditory or sensory warning or recognition by Pt that seizure is imminent.
- Ictal phase (active seizing): Tonic posturing or clonic jerking.
- Postictal phase (after seizure has subsided): AMS, extreme confusion, fatigue, fear, and disorientation.

Create a Safe Environment—Before a Seizure

- Maintain bed in lowest position with side rails raised at all times.
- Install seizure pads to side rails, headboard, and footboard—bath blankets can be used if commercial pads are not available.
- Ensure suction and basic airways (oral or nasal) are readily available at the bedside and in working order.
- Instruct family and visitors on use of call bell.
- Transfer or admit Pt to a room closest to nurse's station.
- Establish an IV in Pts with a known seizure history and whose seizures are known to be frequent or prolonged.

Protect the Pt—During a Seizure

- **If Pt is in bed:** Lower head of bed and raise side rails. Place pillows or blankets between Pt and rails if seizure pads have not already been installed, and call for help.
- **If Pt is out of bed:** Assist Pt to floor, protect from injury by placing pillow or something soft under Pt's head, clear area of hard or sharp objects (e.g., furniture), and call for help.
- Position Pt on his or her side to facilitate drainage of secretions, and prevent Pt's tongue from obstructing airway.
- Do not attempt to restrain Pt during seizure.
- Do not insert anything into Pt's mouth or attempt to hold open the airway or jaw. An oral airway may be inserted for prolonged seizure or signs of hypoxia (e.g., cyanosis), but do not force airway into place—consider a nasal airway.

Recovery—After the Seizure

- Keep Pts on their side until able to protect their own airway.
- Suction oropharynx to clear secretions as needed.
- Examine for injuries—change bedding and clothing if soiled.
- Stay with Pt and withhold food or drink until fully alert.
- Reorient and reassure Pt—allow Pt to sleep if tired.
- Assess mental status and VS every 15 min.
- Monitor labs (seizure medication levels, blood sugar, etc.).
- Document type of seizure and duration.

Shock: Comparing Different Types and Management

	Anaphylactic (Allergic Reaction)	Cardiogenic (Pump Failure)	Hypovolemic (Low Volume)	Neurogenic (Spinal Shock)	Septic (Septicemia)
Clinical Findings	Dyspnea Bronchospasm Hives, rash Cool, pale skin ↓ BP, ↑ HR Diaphoresis Hypotension Edema, swelling	↓ HR, ↓ BP Weak pulses ↑ Capillary refill Cyanosis Dysrhythmias Dyspnea AMS Cool, moist skin	↓ BP, ↑ HR Weak pulses ↑ Capillary refill Cyanosis Dysrhythmias AMS Cool, moist skin	↓ BP, ↓ HR Bounding pulse Pale, warm, and dry skin Skin possibly flushed	Flushed, warm skin ↑Temp, ↓ UO (late) Vasodilatation (early) Vasoconstriction (late)
Management	Support ABCs Administer SC epinephrine, antihistamines, IV fluids, corticosteroids	Support ABCs Administer CPAP Fluid challenge (250–500 mL) if lungs clear Adjust IV to TKO for pulmonary congestion (rales or crackles) Administer vasopressors	Support ABCs Control bleeding Immobilize c-spine for trauma Elevate legs (unless trauma) Establish 2 large-bore IVs (NS/LR) and titrate to SBP >90 mm Hg	Support ABCs Immobilize cervical spine for trauma Give IV fluids Ensure supine position Administer vasopressors	Support ABCs Give IV fluids Obtain blood cultures Administer antibiotics, vasopressors

Suicidal/Combative Patient

- Ensure the safety of yourself and staff.
- Be aware of items or medical equipment that may be used as a weapon.
- Observe Pt closely for signs of potential violence (e.g., threatening posture, agitation, threatening language, fist clenching, wide-eyed stare).
- Observe pupils (dilated = CNS ↑; constricted = CNS ↓).
- Demonstrate confidence, but avoid arguing or confrontation.
- Maintain a safe distance between yourself and Pt.
- Never allow the Pt to block your exits.
- Restrain Pts who are a danger to themselves or others.

Tachycardia (ACLS)

Clinical Findings

Neuro: Dizziness, light-headedness, anxiety, AMS, restlessness.
Resp: SOB, hyperventilation.
CV: HR >100 bpm, chest discomfort, palpitations, dysrhythmias.
Skin: Coolness and moisture, warmth and flushing, tingling sensation.
GI/GU: Nausea and vomiting.
MS: Weakness, fatigue.

Collaborative Management

- Treatment should not be based on HR alone! If Pt is otherwise asymptomatic (no CP or SOB, stable BP, etc.), implement supportive care measures, notify physician STAT, and search for reversible causes.
- If tachycardia results from anxiety or agitation, reduce external stressors (e.g., noise and bright lights, pain management, adjust room temp).
- Lay Pt flat and elevate foot of bed 10°–15° if Pt is light-headed or faint.
- Obtain STAT order for 12-lead ECG; if Pt is monitored, assess ECG rhythm.
- Assess for associated symptoms (CP, respiratory distress, cyanosis, AMS).
- Obtain and document orthostatic vital signs (each set, 1 min apart) from supine, sitting, and standing positions. Use extreme caution (Pt may pass out) and extra staff or specialty equipment (e.g., standing platform) as needed based on Pt's presentation and tolerance to test. **Note**: An increase in HR or decrease in SBP by 20 points from baseline is positive for orthostatic hypotension.

NCLEX **Unstable Tachycardia, All Types (ACLS 2010)**

- ◎ For SINUS tachycardia, search for and treat CAUSES of tachycardia.
- ◎ If Pt unstable (CP, decreased BP, SOB, or AMS), call a code/notify physician STAT. Pt requires immediate intervention!

1. Turn on defibrillator, attach ECG electrodes, press "synch" button, and verify that R waves are sensed by machine. If QRS complex is too wide for machine to identify R waves, switch to unsynchronized cardioversion (follow steps for manual defibrillation).
2. Sedate when clinical situation permits.
3. It may be necessary to adjust gain until each R wave has a synch marker.
4. Select energy level based on arrhythmia and attempt cardioversion. Delays are normal. Do not release discharge buttons until shock is delivered.

Rhythm	Waveform	Sequence
Narrow—Regular (<0.12 sec)	Biphasic	50–100 J (escalate as needed)
	Monophasic	50 J, 100 J, 200 J, 300 J, 360 J
Narrow—Irregular (<0.12 sec)	Biphasic	120–200 J (escalate as needed)
	Monophasic	200 J, 300 J, 360 J
Wide—Regular (≥0.12 sec)	Biphasic	100–120 J (escalate as needed)
	Monophasic	100 J, 200 J, 300 J, 360 J
Wide—Irregular (≥0.12 sec)	Biphasic	120–200 J (defibrillation dose)
	Monophasic	360 J (defibrillation dose)

- Assess rhythm and refer to appropriate algorithm for treatment. Most defibrillators default back to nonsynchronized mode after each synchronized cardioversion. If subsequent synchronized cardioversion is needed, confirm that defibrillator is in synchronized mode.
- Consider torsade de pointes with all polymorphic VT. If synchronization is delayed and clinical situation is critical, go immediately to unsynchronized cardioversion at 120–200 J biphasic or 360 J monophasic.

NCLEX Stable Tachycardia (ACLS 2010)

Treatment should not be based on HR alone! If Pt is otherwise asymptomatic (no CP or SOB, stable BP, etc.), implement supportive care, notify physician STAT, and search for reversible causes. If Pt becomes unstable, see Unstable Arrhythmias.

Narrow—Complex (<0.12 sec)

- Obtain IV access—12 lead if available.
- **Vagal Maneuvers:** Instruct Pt to cough/bear down.
- **Adenosine:** 6 mg rapid IV push—follow with 20 mL rapid NS flush and elevation of extremity—repeat 12 mg if needed using same rapid-push technique. Maintain Pt in a mild, reverse Trendelenburg.

Wide—Complex (≥0.12 sec)

- Obtain IV access—12 lead if available.
- Consider **adenosine** 6 mg rapid IV push if regular and monomorphic (may be aberrant SVT).
- Consider antiarrhythmic—only one—consult expert:
  - **Procainamide**: 20–50 mg/min IV—stop for arrhythmia suppression, hypotension, QRS duration increase of >50%, or max dose of 17 mg/kg. Infusion maintenance: 1–4 mg/min. Avoid with prolonged QT and CHF.
  - **Amiodarone**: 150 mg IV over 10 min—repeat as needed if VT recurs. Follow by infusion maintenance of 1 mg/min for first 6 hr.
  - **Sotalol**: 100 mg (1.5 mg/kg) IV over 5 min—avoid if QT prolonged.

NCLEX Transfusion Reaction

Clinical Findings

Neuro: Anxiety, restlessness.
Resp: SOB, dyspnea, tachypnea, bronchospasm.
CV: Chest pain, tachycardia, hypotension.
Skin: Urticaria, pruritus, erythema, burning at infusion site.
GI/GU: Nausea, vomiting, diarrhea, hematuria, oliguria, anuria.
MS: Flank, back, or joint pain.
Metabolic: Fever, chills.

Collaborative Management

- Stop transfusion and run normal saline to maintain IV access. ◎ Do NOT use lactated Ringer's (LR) solution. It contains calcium and will clot blood in the tubing.
- Notify health-care provider and blood bank of reaction STAT.
- Recheck Pt ID and blood labels for possible errors.
- Return unused blood product to blood bank for analysis.
- Prepare to administer fluids and ordered medications:
  - **Anaphylaxis**: Epinephrine, antihistamines, corticosteroids.
  - **Febrile, nonhemolytic**: Acetaminophen; if Pt develops chills, cover with blanket unless temp. >102°F.
  - **Hemolytic**: Furosemide, low-dose dopamine.
- Assess urinary catheter for output, color, and clarity of urine. If Pt does not have urinary catheter in place, prepare to insert one for monitoring UO.
- Continue IV fluids to maintain minimum UO of 30 mL/hr.
- Monitor for early detection of any hemodynamic instability (e.g., dysrhythmias, abnormal lab values, CHF).

Assessment—Primary Trauma Survey

Airway Management and Cervical Spine Immobilization

- **Open airway:** Use jaw-thrust method, assign c-spine control.
- Assess for compromise/obstruction.
- Suction airway to clear blood, secretions, and debris.
- Have c-collar applied.

Breathing and Ventilation

- Respirations—presence, rate, depth, quality, and effort.
- Inspect and palpate chest, and auscultate lung fields for diminished or absent breath sounds.
- Manually ventilate with a BVM if breathing inadequate.

Circulation and Hemorrhage Control

- Pulse—presence, quality, regularity.
- Begin chest compressions if no palpable pulse.
- Skin—color, temp, moisture, capillary refill.
- Control hemorrhage with direct pressure.

Disability

- Determine and establish baseline GCS score.
- **Pupils:** PERRL (pupils equal, round, and reactive to light).
- Expose/Environment.
- Remove clothing and assess Pt for injury and hemorrhage.
- Maintain body temp by keeping Pt covered.
- Logroll to inspect and palpate posterior surfaces.
- Immobilize entire body using c-spine collar/long board.

Assessment—Secondary Trauma Survey

Vital Signs

- BP, HR, RR, lung sounds, skin color, and temp.
- Assess every 3–5 min or with any change in Pt status.

SAMPLE History

- Signs and symptoms.
- Allergies or sensitivities to medications.
- Medication (prescription or OTC) taken on a regular basis.
- Past medical or surgical history.
- Last meal eaten or last beverage.
- Events leading up to the injury.

Head-to-Toe Assessment

Head and Face

- Pupils—reassess equality and reactivity to light.
- Contusions, abrasions, lacerations, asymmetry.
- Abnormalities of the eyes, eyelids, ears, mouth, mandible.
- Soft tissue injuries, skull depressions, abnormal mobility.

Neck and Cervical Spine

- Contusions, abrasions, lacerations, deformity.
- Tracheal deviation/jugular vein distention (JVD).
- Tenderness, crepitus, subcutaneous emphysema.

Chest and Lungs

- Contusions, abrasions, lacerations, deformity, paradoxical movement, penetrating or sucking chest wounds, splinting, guarding, sternal retractions, steering wheel bruises.
- Anterior lung fields—diminished/absent breath sounds.
- Tenderness, crepitus, subcutaneous emphysema.

Abdomen

- Distention, contusions, abrasions, lacerations, penetrations, ecchymosis, transverse umbilical contusion (seat belt sign).
- All quadrants—tenderness, guarding, softness, rigidity.

Pelvis and Perineum

- Contusions, abrasions, lacerations, hematoma, ecchymosis.
- Perineal injury/bleeding.
- Pelvic tenderness/instability/limb foreshortening.
- Pelvic fracture—shortened, externally rotated leg.

Back (performed during logroll onto long board)

- Contusions, abrasions, lacerations, penetrations, deformity.
- Spinal tenderness/deformity.
- Posterior lung fields—diminished/absent breath sounds.

Extremities

- Deformity, open fractures, dislocation, lacerations, hematoma, ecchymosis, tenderness, crepitus, abnormal movement.
- **Six Ps**: Pain—Pallor—Pulse—Polar—Paresthesia—Paralysis.
- Distal CSM—assess before and after splinting.

- Reassess GCS score, pupils, and sensory and motor function every 3–5 min or with any change in Pt status.

Special Considerations

Pregnancy

- Immobilize pregnant women (>24 wk) in the left lateral position if possible to avoid compression of the vena cava.

Mechanism of Injury

- **Motor vehicle accidents (MVA):** Direction of impact, speed, condition of vehicle, use of seat belts or airbags, ejection from vehicle, was another passenger from same vehicle killed, delayed transport due to extrication.
- **Falls:** From what height and onto what type of surface?
- **Penetrating trauma:** Weapon, site and depth of injury, underlying organs, caliber/velocity of bullet, associated exit wounds.

Indications for Spinal Immobilization

Neurological Findings

- AMS, GCS <15; unequal or unresponsive pupil(s).
- LOC or loss of memory of incident.
- Neurological deficits/symptoms.

Associated Findings

- Spinal tenderness and/or spinal deformity.
- Distracting injury.
- Communication barrier.
- Alcohol or drug involvement.

Mechanism of Injury

- Fall >10 feet.
- Auto versus pedestrian.
- Penetrating injuries of head, chest, back, abdomen, pelvis.
- Significant blunt force trauma to the head, neck, or back.

Assessment—Revised Trauma Score (RTS)

Component	Parameter	Score
Respiratory Rate	10–29/min .4 >29/min .3 6–9/min .2 1–5/min .1 Apnea 0	
SBP	>89 . . . . .4 76–89 . . . . .3 50–75 . . . . .2 1–49 . . . . .1 Pulseless 0	
GCS Score (see p. 61)	13–15 . . . . .4 9–12 . . . . .3 6–8 . . . . .2 4–5 . . . . .1 3 0	
	Total	

Trauma—Basic Management

- Establish and manage ABCs with full c-spine precautions.
- Administer high-flow O_2 or assist ventilations manually.
- Control external bleeding with direct pressure.
- Maintain normal body temp.
- Assess need for advanced airway, and intubate as indicated.
- Start two large-bore IVs titrated to SBP >90 mm Hg.
- Attach ECG monitor and manage dysrhythmias.
- Determine need for transfer to appropriate trauma center.

◎ Watch for abnormal respiratory patterns, changes in LOC and pupils, s/s of increasing ICP, seizures, and posturing.

- Assess pupils and establish a baseline AVPU or GCS.
- Inspect ears for blood and CSF leak; allow nosebleed to drain if CSF leak is present—protect airway and suction as needed.
- Check blood glucose level with all AMS.

Chest Trauma

◎ Watch for respiratory distress, shock, JVD, sub-Q emphysema.

- **Flail chest:** Unstable segment of ribs, paradoxical movement with respiration—stabilize flail segment with bulky dressing.
- **Impaled object:** Stabilize in place with 4 × 4 and tape. Do not remove object unless it interferes with resuscitation.
- **Open/sucking chest wound:** Three-sided, occlusive dressing—if tension pneumothorax develops, remove dressing.
- **Tension pneumothorax:** Respiratory distress, absent breath sounds on affected side, and/or tracheal deviation. Definitive care includes immediate needle decompression on affected side.

Chest Trauma Comparing Different Types

	Pneumothorax	Hemothorax	Tamponade
Impression	Respiratory distress		Shock
Heart	Normal sound	Can be muffled	Muffled
Lungs	Diminished on affected side		Normal
Trachea	Shifted away	May be shifted	Midline
Neck Veins	Distended	Distended	Distended
Percussion	Hyperresonant	Dull	Normal

Abdominal Trauma

◎ Watch for guarding, bruising, rigidity, distension, or hypotension. Anticipate internal hemorrhage.

Impaled objects

- Secure in place with 4 × 4 and tape.
- Do not remove object unless it interferes with resuscitation.

Eviscerations

- Cover with saline-soaked, sterile gauze dressing.
- Do not inflate abdominal compartment if using pneumatic antishock garment (PASG).
- Do not place organs back into abdominal cavity.

Extremity Trauma

- Immobilize extremity in place.
- Assess distal CSM (circulation, sensory and motor function) before and after immobilization. Leave fingertips and toes exposed.
- Do not attempt to reduce fractures.
- Cover any exposed bone with saline-soaked, sterile gauze dressing.
- Apply traction splint to midshaft femur fractures.
- Paramedics may apply PASG in the field to splint lower extremity fractures (use varies by region).
- Consider morphine (2–4 mg IV) or fentanyl (25–50 mcg IV) for moderate-to-severe pain (for isolated extremity injury only).
- Pt meets criteria for critical trauma with two or more long-bone fractures or any amputation proximal to wrist or ankle.

Amputations

- Manage life-threatening injuries first!
- Irrigate debris from amputated part with saline.
- Wrap part in gauze moistened with saline (avoid soaking gauze, which causes tissue to macerate and diminishes viability [especially digits]).
- Place wrapped part into a ziplock bag (note time on bag) and then place sealed bag into a container of ice water.
- Immobilize partial amputations in anatomical position.

Abuse

NCLEX Abusive Partner (Domestic Violence)

- Often, battered partners minimize injuries or seriousness of situation.
- Repeated visits to ED with increasing severity of injuries.
- Overprotective partner who refuses to leave Pt alone with staff.
- Signs of trauma consistent with physical and sexual assault.

NCLEX Child Abuse/Neglect

- Unlikely mechanism of injury (story not matching injury).
- Details of injury changing from person to person.
- Burns (scalding or cigarettes) or wire marks.
- Fractures or dislocations in a child <2 yr old.
- Multiple injuries in various stages of healing.
- Unexcused delay in seeking medical attention.
- History inconsistent with child's developmental stages.
- Overly protective parent (interferes with assessment).
- Unusual fear of parent or desire to please parent.
- Withdrawn or aggressive behavior.
- Malnutrition, insect infestation, or disheveled appearance.

NCLEX Elder Abuse/Neglect

- Malnourishment and unexplained dehydration.
- Poor hygiene (body/clothing soiled with urine and feces).
- Clothing inappropriate for weather/season.
- Inappropriate use of restraints (bruising/abrasions of wrists and ankles).

NCLEX Sexual Abuse (Child Molestation)

- Bruised or bleeding genitalia or blood-stained underwear.
- Painful urination or itching of genital area.
- STD or pregnancy.
- Inappropriate display of sexual behavior.

Collaborative Management

- Remove victim from abusive environment.
- Avoid any confrontation with alleged abuser.
- Avoid examining genitalia except to control hemorrhage.
- Sexual assault victims should be seen at a facility with staff trained and equipped for examining and collecting sexual assault evidence; they should not bathe, douche, urinate, or change clothes before being examined.
- Notify appropriate authorities or protective services when abuse is suspected.

Emergency Management for All Pts

- Follow standard protocol for supporting ABCs.
- Carefully remove any remaining, visible venom apparatus.*
- Keep Pt warm and calm, and avoid excessive movement.
- Apply cold compress**/sterile dressing to affected area.
- Remove rings and constricting jewelry from affected area.
- Immobilize extremity with loose splint to restrict movement.
- Keep affected area below level of heart.
- Attempt to identify insect or animal for correct antidote.
- Manage allergic reaction/anaphylaxis (see pp. 128–129).

Arachnid (Spiders) and Scorpions

Black widow

- **Classic presentation**: Abdominal rigidity and pain, HA, dizziness, shoulder and backache, n/v, sweating, and salivation.
- Increased morbidity and mortality in very young children and the elderly.

Brown recluse

- Spider identified by a violin-shaped pattern on back.
- **Tell-tale sign**: Reddish ulcer surrounded by a whitish blue "bull's-eye."
- Other than an inconspicuous bite mark, s/s usually won't show for 24 hr.

Scorpion

- Bark scorpion (southwestern United States) is the only lethal species in the U.S.
- Anticipate shock—support ABCs.

Hymenoptera (Bees, Wasps, and Ants)

- ***Remove stingers by scraping only!** Avoid tweezers, because squeezing venom sac will only inject more venom.
- If Pt has Epi-Pen, assist with administration.

Snake Envenomation

- Anticipate shock—support ABCs.
- Avoid practices such as tourniquets or excision and suction.
- ****Do not use cold compresses or ice on affected area.**

Marine Animals

Jelly Fish/Sea Anemones (Tentacles)

- Carefully remove visible tentacles or spines. Irrigate skin with 5% acetic acid (household vinegar), isopropanol, or seawater. Do not use freshwater.

- Carefully remove spines if possible and immerse affected area in water as warm as Pt can tolerate without scalding (<110°F/42°C).

Burn Injury

Degree	Burn Depth/Penetration	Appearance
First	Epidermis only	Sunburn-like, no blistering
Second	Epidermis + partial dermis	Blistering
Third	Dermis + underlying tissue (full thickness)	Eschar and/or whitish gray appearance

Burn Assessment

- TBSA (total body surface area): count only 2nd- and 3rd-degree burns.
- Age of Pt (age + TBSA = % probability of mortality).
- Pulmonary injury (smoke inhalation, toxic fumes).
- Associated injuries (airway burns and other trauma).
- Chemical/electrical burns, carbon monoxide poisoning.
- Pre-existing diseases (potential for exacerbation).

Collaborative Management

- Anticipate laryngospasm/airway complications.
- Anticipate and prepare for transfer to a burn center.
- Initiate fluid resuscitation as ordered.

Fluid Resuscitation—First 24 hr (start from time of injury)

Indications

- Adults with 2nd- or 3rd-degree burns >20% of TBSA.
- Children >1 yr with 2nd- or 3rd-degree burns ≥15% TBSA.
- All infants with 2nd- or 3rd-degree burns of ≥10% TBSA.

NCLEX *Management (Parkland Formula)*

- 4 mL × kg × %TBSA burned (2nd-degree + 3rd-degree burn injury).
- Infuse half over the first 8 hr (from time of burn).
- Infuse the remaining half over the next 16 hr.

NCLEX

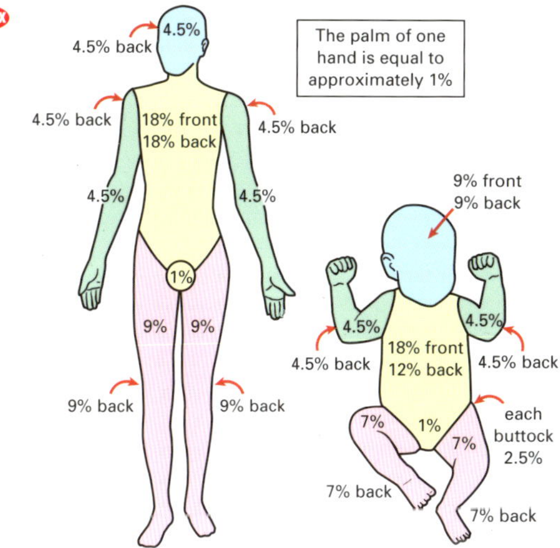

Clinical Findings

- **General:** White, waxy, mottled appearance, loss of sensation.
- **First-degree:** Erythema, edema, waxy, hard white plaques.
- **Second-degree:** Formation of clear blisters within 24 hr.
- **Third-degree:** Formation of blood-filled blisters.
- **Fourth-degree:** Full-thickness (muscle, tendons, and bones).
- **Thawing:** Red, warm, edema, burning, stinging, painful.

Collaborative Management

- Remove Pt from cold environment.
- Remove wet clothing, and protect Pt from further heat loss or hypothermia.
- Anticipate and manage hypothermia per protocol.
- Avoid excessive or rough handling of Pt or affected area.
- Do not massage frostbitten area.
- Leave blisters intact.
- Remove jewelry and keep affected area slightly elevated.
- For first-degree injury—position Pt with affected area against warm body surface (e.g., placing frostbitten fingers into the axilla).
- Encourage warm, nonalcoholic beverage unless AMS or trauma present.
- Monitor ECG and manage dysrhythmias per hypothermia protocol.
- Obtain IV access in a nonfrostbitten extremity.
- Consider **Morphine** 1–4 mg IV or **Fentanyl** 25–50 mcg IV for pain.

Rapid Thawing Procedure

- Caution: Avoid thawing procedures if refreezing is likely.
- Submerse affected area in warm water (38°–42°C/102°–108°F) for 10–30 min (may use warm wet packs).
- Carefully separate digits with cotton or gauze.
- Elevate extremity slightly to minimize swelling.
- Manage pain as needed.

Drowning—Near Drowning—Submersion

Collaborative Management

- Bathtub and bucket drowning—consider child abuse.
- Note length of time Pt in water, water temp, and whether freshwater or salt water.
- Obtain quick history (diving or boating accident, alcohol, etc.).
- Establish and manage ABCs per protocol.
- Administer high-flow O_2 via NRB mask or provide PPVs or CPAP if indicated.
- Remove wet garments, and protect Pt against further heat loss.

- Anticipate and manage hypothermia and associated traumatic injuries.
- Attach ECG monitor and manage dysrhythmias per ACLS.*

Special Considerations

- ***Cold Water Submersion**: A Pt's chance of survival may increase significantly if the submersion event occurs in cold water; therefore, resuscitation should continue while aggressive attempts are implemented to restore normal core temp. Withhold drugs until core temp is >30°C.

Scuba Diving—Decompression Sickness (DCS)

- **S/S**: Joint pain, AMS, fatigue, visual disturbances, increased RR and HR, hypotension, n/v, cyanosis, and seizure activity.
- Manage ABCs normally.
- Do not place Pt in Trendelenburg position (increases ICP).
- Transfer to facility with hyperbaric oxygen capabilities.
- Consider aspirin for potential blood coagulation disorder.
- Needle chest decompression for tension pneumothorax.

High-Altitude Illness

Acute Mountain Sickness (AMS)

- Most common at or above 2500 meters (8200 ft).
- **S/S**: Fatigue, lethargy, anorexia, n/v, insomnia, dizziness, increased HR or RR (progresses to HACE, see next section).
- **Management**: ABCs, O_2, descent, supportive care.

High Altitude Cerebral Edema (HACE)

- Most common at or above 4800 meters (15,750 ft).
- **S/S**: (severe AMS) Ataxia and/or an altered mental status in addition to any one of the signs of AMS.
- **Management**: ABCs, immediate descent, O_2, hyperbaric therapy (Gamow Bag/Tent). Consider Decadron 8 mg IM, IV.

High Altitude Pulmonary Edema (HAPE)

- Most common at or above 4500 m (14,700 ft).
- **S/S**: Dyspnea, SOB, crackles, cyanosis, dry cough (progresses to pink, frothy sputum), tachycardia, tachypnea, mild fever.
- **Management**: ABCs, descent, O_2, CPAP, rewarming, hyperbaric therapy. Consider nifedipine 10 mg PO.
- Can also occur in residents of high altitude who travel to low altitude and then return to altitude (re-ascent HAPE).

Differentiating Heatstroke and Heat Exhaustion

	Heatstroke	Heat Exhaustion
Core Temp	>104°F (40°C)	<104°F (40°C)
Skin	Dry, hot, flushed (late), can be moist (early on)	Profuse sweating
Neuro	Significant AMS	Fatigue, HA, agitation
S/s common to both	Tachypnea, nausea and vomiting, tachycardia, weakness, fatigue, dehydration, hypotension	

Collaborative Management

- Remove Pt from heat source and loosen or remove clothing.
- Establish and manage ABCs per protocol.
- Administer high-flow O_2 or manually ventilate as indicated.
- Obtain baseline VS including core temp.
- Begin rapid cooling measures if indicated.
- Obtain finger-stick blood glucose level.
- Position supine with feet elevated if exhibiting s/s of shock.
- Attach ECG monitor and manage dysrhythmias per ACLS.
- Obtain IV access and bolus with 500–1000 mL NS.

Rapid Cooling Measures

- Indicated for a core temp >104°F (40°C).
- Remove clothing from Pt if not already done.
- Use a fan to increase airflow over disrobed Pt while misting with warm water (warm water helps to prevent shivering).
- Place ice packs to axilla and groin.
- Diazepam or lorazepam will help to suppress shivering.
- Caution: To avoid the risk of hypothermia, stop cooling measure once core temp has reached 102°F (39°C).

Hypothermia

Initial Therapy for All Patients

- Establish and maintain ABCs per protocol.
- Remove wet garments, and protect Pt against further heat loss.
- Monitor core temp and cardiac rhythm.
- Manage dysrhythmias. Note: Watch for tachycardia (early), bradycardia (late), and J waves.

Pulse and Breathing Present	No Pulse or Respiration
34°–36°C (mild) • Passive rewarming. • Active external rewarming.	• Initiate CPR. • Defibrillate VF/VT: biphasic 200 J; monophasic 360 J. • Intubate and confirm placement. • Ventilate with warm, humidified O_2 (42°–46°C). • Establish IV and infuse warm normal saline (43°C).
30°—34°C (moderate) • Passive rewarming. • Active external rewarming of truncal areas only.	**Core temp <30°C** • Continue CPR, withhold drugs, limit to one shock for VF/VT. • Active internal rewarming sequence.
<30°C (severe hypothermia) • Active internal rewarming sequence. • Continue rewarming until a core temp of >35°C is achieved or return of spontaneous circulation or resuscitative efforts cease.	**Core temp >30°C** • Continue CPR. • Drugs as indicated, but spaced longer apart. • Repeat shocks for VF/VT as core temp rises. • Active internal rewarming.

Active Internal Rewarming

- Warm IV fluids (43°C)
- Warm humid oxygen (42°—46°C)
- Peritoneal lavage (use only potassium-free fluid)
- Extracorporeal rewarming

Hazmat/Weapons of Mass Destruction (WMD)

Type of Incident	Agency	Phone Number
Biological Agents	CDC 24-hr	770-488-7100
	USAMRIID	888-872-7443
Chemical/Hazmat	CHEMTREC	800-424-9300
Radiation Release	REAC/TS	423-576-3131

Protect yourself first!

Organophosphate (OPP)/Carbamate Exposure

- Remove from source, and remove Pt's clothing and jewelry.
- Decontaminate with copious NS or water.
- **Atropine**: 2–5 mg (**Peds**: 0.05 mg/kg) IV, IM repeated every 3–5 min until signs of SLUDGEM resolve.
- **Pralidoxime* (2-PAM)**: 600 mg IM or may infuse 1–2 g over 15–30 min (**Peds**: 20–50 mg/kg IM or infuse over 15–30 min). *Not recommended for carbamates!
- Do not induce vomiting if substance is ingested! If Pt alert with gag reflex, give water 5 mL/kg (max 200 mL) PO.

Carbon Monoxide Exposure

- Remove from source and remove clothing.
- High-flow oxygen.
- Rapid transport for hyperbaric therapy.

Cyanide Exposure

- See Chemical and Nerve Agents (p. 162).
- Extricate Pt, remove clothing and jewelry, support ABCs.
- **Hydroxocobalamin**: 5 g (**Peds**: 70 mg/kg) IV infused over 15 min or **Cyanide Antidote Kit**.

Hydrocarbon (Methylene Chlorido, Xylene) Exposure

- Common in inhalation (huffing/sniffing) of aerosol fumes.
- Remove from source and remove clothing.
- Do not induce vomiting if substance is ingested!
- Decontaminate with copious NS or water.

Ammonia or Chlorine Exposure

- Remove from source and remove clothing.
- Decontaminate with copious NS or water.
- Manage pulmonary edema per standard protocol.

Caustic (Acids and Alkalis) Exposure

- Remove from source and remove clothing.
- **Solid (powder) corrosive**: Brush off dry particles.
- **Liquid corrosive**: Decontaminate with copious NS or water.
- Do not induce vomiting if substance is ingested! If Pt alert with gag reflex, give **water or milk**: 200–300 mL (**Peds**: 15 mL/kg).

Biological Agents

Anthrax (Inhalation, Cutaneous)

- **S/S**: Inhalation: Initial flu-like symptoms—progresses to severe respiratory difficulty and shock. Cutaneous: marked by a boil-like lesion that forms an ulcer with a black center.
- **Exposure Risk**: Low—Inhalation anthrax cannot be transmitted from person to person (cutaneous anthrax can but is rare).
- **Treatment**: Use standard precautions, support ABCs.

Botulism

- **S/S**: Progressive, descending muscle weakness that leads to full-body paralysis and respiratory failure, drooping eyelids, slurred speech, difficulty swallowing, dry mouth.
- **Exposure Risk**: None—not spread from person to person.
- **Treatment**: Use standard precautions, support ABCs. Botulinum antitoxin—prehospital use not recommended.

Hemorrhagic Fevers (Ebola, Hanta, Marburg, etc.)

- **S/S**: Early—High fever, HA, fatigue, abdominal pain; Late—hematemesis, diarrhea, rash, bleeding mucous membranes.
- **Exposure Risk**: High—Transmitted from person to person or from contaminated surface to person.
- **Treatment**: Use contact precautions, support ABCs. Antibiotics—doxycycline or ciprofloxacin given in hospital.

Plague

- **S/S**: Fever, cough, chest pain, hemoptysis.
- **Exposure Risk**: High—Pts are contagious until they have completed 72 hr of antibiotic treatment.
- **Treatment**: Use droplet precautions and support ABCs. Antibiotics—doxycycline or ciprofloxacin given in hospital.

Smallpox

- **S/S**: Skin lesions (pox)—more prominent on the head and extremities, and lesions all appear to be of the same age. (Chicken pox is concentrated around the trunk, and lesions appear to be in different stages of healing.)
- **Exposure Risk**: High—From onset of rash until lesions have scabbed over and fallen off (approximately 3 wk).
- **Treatment**: Airborne/contact precautions, ABCs.

Vesicants (Mustard Gas, Lewisite, Phosgene)

- **S/S**: Erythema, blistering, burning, itching and stinging of skin, tearing and burning of eyes, sore throat, productive cough, laryngitis, irritated, bloody nose, light sensitivity.
- **Exposure Risk**: High—Avoid contact with agent or fumes.
- **Treatment**: Use maximum PPE, decontamination with copious water, support ABCs. For lewisite (severe cases), BAL (British anti-lewisite) is administered: 3 mg/kg deep IM.

Nerve Agents (Sarin, VX, Soman, Tabun)

- **S/S**: Salivation, lacrimation, urination, defecation, GI upset, emesis, muscle twitching, as well as coma and seizures.
- **Exposure Risk**: High—avoid contact with agent or fumes.
- **Treatment**: Use maximum PPE, remove from source, remove clothing, decontaminate with copious water, and support ABCs aggressively and administer antidote.
- **Mark-I Kit**: Atropine: 2–5 mg (Peds: 0.05 mg/kg) IM every 3–5 min until signs of SLUDGEM resolve; Pralidoxime (2-PAM): 600 mg IM or may infuse 1–2 g over 15–30 min (Peds: 20–50 mg/kg IM or infuse over 15–30 min).
- **Diazepam**: 5–10 mg (Peds: 0.2 mg/kg) IV for seizures.

Pulmonary Agents (Chlorine, Diphosgene, PFIB)

- **S/S**: Eye and nasal irritation, tearing, chest pressure, cough, choking, hemoptysis, rales, pulmonary edema
- **Exposure Risk**: Low—Avoid contact with agent or fumes.
- **Treatment**: Use standard precautions, remove from source, decontaminate with copious water, support ABCs.

Cyanide

- **S/S**: Gasping, flushing, faintness, sweating, confusion, HA, seizure, coma, respiratory/cardiac arrest (cyanosis is rare).
- **Exposure Risk**: Low—Avoid contact with agent or fumes.
- **Treatment**: Remove from source, remove clothing, support ABCs aggressively, and administer antidote.
- **Hydroxocobalamin**: 5 g (Peds: 70 mg/kg) IV infused over 15 min *or*
- **Cyanide Antidote Kit**:
  - **Amyl nitrite**: 1 ampule crushed and inhaled every minute until IV established; *then*
  - **Sodium nitrite**: 300 mg over 5 min; *then*
  - **Sodium thiosulfate**: 12.5 g IV over 5 min.

Abbreviation Alert!

Joint Commission Official “Do Not Use” List: 2009

Do Not Use	Rationale	Use Instead
U (unit)	Mistaken for “0” (zero), the number “4” or “cc”	Write “unit”
IU (international unit)	Mistaken for “IV” (intravenous) or the number “10” (ten)	Write “international unit”
Q.D., QD, q.d., qd (daily) Q.O.D., QOD, q.o.d., qod (every other day)	Mistaken for each other Period after the Q mistaken for “I” and the “O” mistaken for “I”	Write “daily” Write “every other day”
Trailing zero (X.0 mg)* Lack of leading zero (.X mg)	Decimal point is missed	Write X mg Write 0.X mg
MS MSO_4 and $MgSO_4$	Confused for one another Can mean morphine sulfate or magnesium sulfate	Write “morphine sulfate” Write “magnesium sulfate”

*Exception: A “trailing zero” may be used only where required to demonstrate level of precision of value being reported (e.g., catheter tube sizes). It may not be used in medication-related documentation.

Additional Abbreviations, Acronyms, and Symbols

Do Not Use	Rationale	Use Instead
> (greater than) < (less than)	Misinterpreted as the number “7” (seven) or the letter “L” Confused with one another	Write “greater than” Write “less than”
Abbreviated drug names	Misinterpreted because of similar abbreviations for multiple drugs	Write drug names in full
Apothecary units	Unfamiliar to many practitioners Confused with metric units	Use metric units
@	Mistaken for the number “2” (two)	Write “at”

cc	Mistaken for "U" (units) when poorly written	Write "mL" or "ml" or "milliliters" ("mL" is preferred)
µg	Mistaken for mg (milligrams) resulting in 1000-fold overdose	Write "mcg" or "micrograms"

Administration Alerts!

Always Remember! Assessment and Documentation

- Assessment needs vary and depend on route and medication.
- Assess Pt and record VS before and after giving drugs that may adversely affect RR, HR, BP, LOC, and blood glucose, and monitor labs as indicated.
- Evaluate meds for their effectiveness and for ADR to drugs not previously taken by Pt.
- Verify allergies and assess for reactions to drugs not previously taken by Pt.
- Document drug, dose, route, time given, discontinue (d/c) time if applicable, Pt's response, and any ADR.

Always Remember! Critical General Points

- NCLEX Confirm MAR is up to date, and question unclear medication orders.
- Follow institution policy regarding double-checking certain high-risk medications (e.g., heparin, insulin) and pediatric dosages.
- Confirm compatibility if Pt is taking multiple medications.
- Do not crush sustained-release or enteric-coated capsules or pills.
- Always use filter needle to withdraw medication from glass ampule. Discard and replace filter needle with regular injection needle before injection.
- Use straw for liquid PO iron to prevent staining of Pt's teeth.

Always Remember! Medication Right

Right Pt
Right Medication
Right Dose
Right Time
Right Route
Right Documentation

Always Remember! Triple Check

FIRST: When obtaining medication—before opening pill packaging or drawing drug up from a vial/ampule.

SECOND: Side-by-side comparison of medication and written order and MAR while preparing drug.

THIRD: After preparation, just before administration at Pt's bedside—identify Pt and verify Pt's name band matches medication order.

Administration Routes

◎ Always refer to Administration Alerts!

Buccal—Transmucosal

1. Offer water to moisten mucous membranes if dry; if on fluid restrictions, Pt can swish and spit.
2. Don gloves and place medication between cheek and gum on either side of Pt's mouth. Avoid areas with inflammation or bleeding.
3. Instruct Pt to allow medication to dissolve: Do not chew or swallow.

Ears—Drops

1. **Position:** Side lying or sitting with head tilted to the side.
2. Gently grasp the rigid, upper cartilage of external ear (auricle).
3. Pts >3 years: Pull auricle upward and back.
4. Pts ≤ 3 years: Pull lobe downward and back.
5. Administer prescribed drops in ear, being careful not to allow dropper tip to touch Pt's ear.
6. Release ear and clean off any excess medication from around the outside of the Pt's ear.
7. Pt should maintain position for 3–5 min.

Note: AD = right ear; AS = left ear; AU = both ears.

Eyes—Drops or Ointment

1. **Position:** Upright with head tilted back slightly.
2. Stand so that dominant hand is toward Pt's forehead.
3. Wipe excessive tearing or drainage from lower eyelid as needed. Use a separate tissue or cotton ball for each eye, and wipe from inner to outer

5. Position heel of dominant hand on Pt's forehead.
6. Use a cotton ball and your nondominant hand to gently pull lower eyelid down. Instruct Pt to look toward forehead.
7. Administer prescribed drops into conjunctival sack (apply ointment from inner to outer canthus), being careful not to allow dropper tip or ointment applicator tip to touch Pt.
8. Instruct Pt to gently close eyes for 1–2 min.

Note: OD = right eye; OS = left eye; OU = both eyes.

Inhalation—Handheld Nebulizer

1. **Position:** Sitting upright as tolerated.
2. Pour prescribed volume of medication into nebulizer reservoir.
3. Assemble nebulizer—place cap over reservoir, attach T-piece to cap, attach large tube and mouthpiece to both ends of T-piece, attach oxygen tubing to bottom of reservoir, and connect tubing to oxygen or compressed air source. Clinical tip: A simple mask can be used by removing oxygen tubing connector and connecting nebulizer cap directly to mask.
4. Adjust oxygen flow rate to 6–8 LPM, or as ordered. Note that lower flow rates produce larger (heavier) droplets that tend to settle in the upper airways; higher flow rates produce smaller (lighter) droplets that are ideal for infiltrating the smaller, lower airways.
5. Instruct Pt to take slow, deep breathes with lips sealed tightly around mouthpiece. Explain need to maintain nebulizer in an upright position.
6. Therapy is complete when misting stops, usually after about 6–8 min. Tap side of reservoir to dislodge any remaining medication.

Inhalation—Metered Dose Inhaler

1. **Position:** Upright as tolerated.
2. Shake inhalers that contain liquid medication; attach spacer if using.
3. Instruct Pt to tilt head back slightly, seal lips around mouthpiece and exhale completely.
4. Administer medication—press down on inhaler as Pt begins to inhale. Encourage Pt to inhale deeply and slowly.
5. ◎ Do not shake powered inhalants, such as Advair, before administration.

Injection

See pp. 172–177.

IV

See pp. 180–181.

Nasogastric—Gastric Tubes

1. **Position:** Semi-Fowler's position if in bed or sitting upright if in chair.
2. Place absorbent pad over Pt's chest beneath NG tube.
3. Prepare medication—pill(s): Crush using a mortar and pestle, pill crusher, or between two spoons; capsule(s): open and empty contents into medicine cup.

◎ Never crush sustained-release or enteric-coated pills; liquid medication is preferred to ensure more accurate dosing.

4. Mix with 10–20 mL of warm water.
5. Unclamp NG tube and confirm proper placement (p. 21).
6. Flush NG tube with 30 mL of water.
7. Draw up and administer prepared medication.
8. Flush NG tube with 30 mL of water.
9. Clamp NG tube for 30 min and instruct Pt to remain upright for 30–45 min.

◎ Do not mix medications with tube-feeding formula.

Oral (PO)

1. **Position:** Upright as tolerated.
2. Offer water or juice as permitted. Pt may prefer med cup to handling medication with his or her hands.
3. Observe Pt until all medication is swallowed: Never leave medication at Pt's bedside.
4. Use straw for liquid PO iron to prevent staining of Pt's teeth.

Rectal (PR)

1. **Position:** Side lying with knees flexed (left lateral preferred). Drape Pt as needed for privacy. Consider placing absorbent pad beneath Pt's hips.
2. Don gloves and lubricate rounded end of suppository with water-soluble lubricant.
3. Spread buttocks and gently insert rounded end of suppository into rectum to the full length of your finger.
4. Instruct Pts to squeeze buttocks together for 3–5 min and to remain on their side for 15–20 min.

Sublingual

1. Offer water to moisten mucous membranes if dry. If on fluid restrictions, Pt can swish and spit.
2. Don gloves and place medication under Pt's tongue. Avoid areas with inflammation or bleeding.
3. Instruct Pt to allow medication to dissolve and not to chew or swallow.

Topical

Intact Skin

1. Don nonsterile gloves if skin is intact or sterile gloves if incision or open wound is present.
2. Unless contraindicated, wash area with warm, soapy water and blot dry.

Nonintact Skin (Incision or Open Wound)

1. Don sterile gloves and use sterile technique.
2. Unless contraindicated, wash area with sterile cleansing solution, and blot dry with sterile gauze.

Creams, Gels, Lotions, Ointments

1. Don gloves.
2. Squeeze (or pour) onto fingertips and apply to area with a gentle massaging motion until medication is absorbed. Refer to medication package for application-specific instructions.
3. Use a sterile tongue depressor if obtaining medication from a multidose container.

Nitroglycerin

◎ Avoid skin contact with nitroglycerin ointment or paste.

1. Wash off old nitroglycerin with warm soap and water and blot dry.
2. Squeeze ordered number of inches onto ruled application paper supplied with the nitroglycerin. Use plastic wrap alternatively.
3. Apply to upper chest or upper arm (area with least amount of hair). Secure application paper/plastic wrap with tape.

Sprays

1. Apply light coat to area. Refer to packaging for instructions.
2. If spray to be applied to chest or above, instruct Pt to close eyes and look away during application, and to gently cover nose and mouth with clean gauze.

Transdermal Patch

1. Don gloves to avoid contact with medication when applying (or removing) patch. Discard old patch per institutional policy.
2. Choose appropriate site: Skin should be intact, clean and dry, free of irritation or breakdown, and free of hair.
3. If replacing old patch, clean and dry site with washcloth and warm soap and water. Rotate sites whenever possible.
4. Write date and time on patch just before application.
5. Remove adhesive backing and apply patch. Hold, applying gentle pressure with palm or finger for 10 sec—do not massage.

Vaginal (PV)

1. **Position:** Supine with knees flexed. Drape Pt as needed for privacy. Consider placing absorbent pad beneath Pt's hips.
2. Don gloves.
3. Spread labia and clean vaginal opening with a warm washcloth, wiping front to back. Use a different corner for each wipe.
4. Discard and replace gloves.

Applicator

1. Fill applicator with prescribed amount of cream and lubricate applicator with water-soluble lubricant.
2. Spread labia and gently insert applicator (using a rolling motion) downward toward sacrum; insert full length of applicator unless resistance is met.
3. Release labia and administer the full amount of cream. Remove applicator (with plunger depressed) and dispose in biohazard container.

Suppository

1. Lubricate rounded end of suppository with water-soluble lubricant.
2. Spread labia and gently insert rounded end of suppository along posterior wall of vagina to the full length of your finger.
3. Instruct Pt to remain supine for 5–10 min.
4. Provide Pt with perineal pad to absorb drainage.

Administration—Preparation

Ampule

◎ Always use a filter needle or a filter straw when drawing up medication from an ampule.

1. Gently shake or flick top of ampule to ensure all medication is at bottom of

unopened alcohol swab with other hand.
3. Snap top of ampule off—away from yourself.
4. Tilt ampule, insert filter needle into liquid, and withdraw desired amount of medication plus an additional 0.2–0.5 mL of air. Avoid touching rim of ampule with filter needle.
5. Remove and discard filter needle, and replace it with needle intended for injection.
6. Expel air until desired volume of medication remains in syringe.

Vial

◎ Needleless (harpoon-type) vial access devices can be used only on single-use vials.

1. Clean rubber top of vial with an alcohol swab or alcohol-based 4% chlorhexidine wipe. Cleaning is not necessary if opening a brand-new, unused vial for first use.
2. Draw air into syringe equal to amount to be withdrawn from vial.
3. Insert needle or vial access device at a 45° angle with bevel up and bring needle upright to 90° as you penetrate rubber top—prevents coring of rubber top.
4. Position needle tip above fluid level and inject air.
5. Invert vial and slowly withdraw medication—keep syringe vertical.
6. Tap base of syringe to move air bubbles to hub of syringe.
7. Inject and withdraw medication as needed until correct dose is obtained and no air remains in syringe.
8. Confirm correct dose of medication and withdraw needle.

Formulas: Medication and Infusion Rates

IV Push and PO Liquid How much solution to draw up	$\frac{\text{Dose Ordered} \times \text{Total Volume}}{\text{Total Amount on Hand}}$
Pills or Tablets: How many pills or tablets May need to be scored	$\frac{\text{Dose Ordered}}{\text{Amount per Pill}}$
Infusion of Volume Only (e.g., 150 mL/hr)	$\frac{\text{Volume/hr} \times \text{Drip Set Factor}}{\text{Time (min)}}$
Infusion of Medication (e.g., 20 mg/hr or 20 mg/kg/hr)	$\frac{\frac{\text{Dose} \times \text{Weight} \times \text{Volume}}{\text{Total Amount on Hand}} \times \text{Drip Set Factor}}{\text{Time (min)}}$
Determine Rate of Existing IV	$\frac{\text{Drops/min} \times 60}{\text{Drip Set Factor}}$

IV Fluid Drip Rate Table (drops/min)*

IV Drip Set	Rate (mL/hr)								
	30	50	75	100	125	150	175	200	250
10 drops/mL	5	8	13	17	21	25	29	33	42
12 drops/mL	6	10	15	20	25	30	35	40	50
15 drops/mL	8	13	19	25	31	37	44	50	62
20 drops/mL	10	17	25	33	42	50	58	67	83
60 drops/mL	30	50	75	100	125	150	175	200	250

***Note:** TKO is 30–60 mL/hr. For microdrip tubing, mL/hr is equal to drops/min.

High-Alert Medication Classes

- Adrenergic agonists/antagonists
- Anesthetic agents
- Cardioplegic solutions
- Chemotherapeutic agents
- Dextrose solutions >20%
- Dialysis solutions
- Epidural/intrathecal meds
- Glycoprotein IIb/IIIa inhibitors
- Hypoglycemic agents (oral)
- Inotropic meds
- Liposomal forms of drugs
- Moderate sedatives
- Narcotics and opiates
- Neuromuscular blocking agents
- Radiocontrast agents
- Saline solutions >0.9%
- Thrombolytics and fibrinolytics
- TPN solutions

Specific High-Alert Medications

- Insulin (IV and SC)
- Amiodarone (IV)
- Calcium (IV)
- Colchicine (IV)
- Digoxin (IV)
- Heparin (IV)
- Lidocaine (IV)
- Magnesium (IV)
- Nitroprusside (IV)
- Potassium (IV)
- Methotrexate
- Nesiritide
- Warfarin

Used with permission from the Institute for Safe Medication Practices. Report medication errors or near misses to the ISMP Medication Errors Reporting Program (MERP)

Injections

	ID	IM	SC
Site	Inner forearm Alternate sites: upper posterior arm, chest and upper back	Deltoid, ventrogluteal, and vastus lateralis ◎ Dorsogluteal no longer recommended	Upper posterior arm, upper back, low back, anterior or lateral thigh and abdomen
Gauge	27–30 g	23 g	25–28 g
Length	1/4–3/8″	1–1 1/2″	3/8–5/8″
Angle	10°–15°	90°	90° or 45° for very thin Pts
Volume	0.1–0.2 mL	≤3 mL; small muscles (deltoid) maximum 1 mL	0.5–1 mL

Angle of Injection

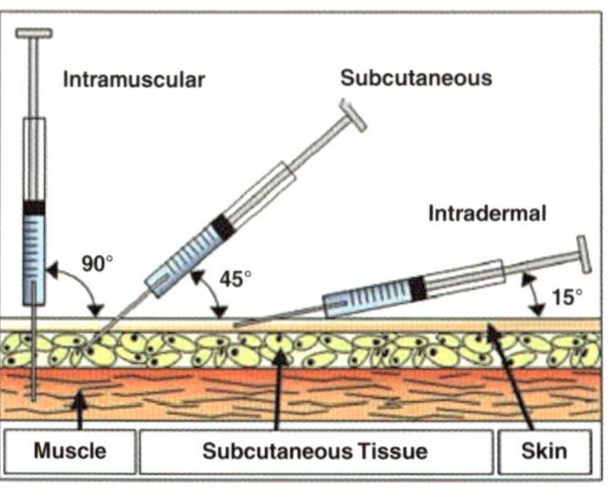

Injections—Intradermal (ID)

1. Select site; inner aspect of forearm is most common.
2. Position Pt, arm supported, forearm facing up.
3. Don gloves.
4. Cleanse site with antiseptic using moderate friction in a circular motion, moving outward from injection site. Avoid touching injection site once prepared.
5. Apply traction. Stretch skin toward hand opposite direction of needle.
6. Insert needle bevel side up just below skin at 10°–15°.
7. Continue to advance needle another 1–2 mm.
8. Inject medication slowly until a small wheal (raised area) appears. A well-defined wheal indicates injection into ID tissue; lack of a wheal indicates injection into SC tissue.
9. Remove needle quickly at same angle as injection.
10. If indicated, mark area around the wheal with a pen.

Injections—Intramuscular (IM)

1. Position Pt according to injection site. Site selection is based on Pt's age and size and the quantity to be injected.
2. Don gloves.
3. Cleanse site with antiseptic using moderate friction in a circular motion, moving outward from injection site. Avoid touching injection site once prepped.
4. Landmark the site. Spread thumb and index finger (nondominant hand) apart, forming a V over injection site, pulling skin taut.
5. Insert needle at a 90° angle with a quick, smooth motion.
6. Stabilize syringe with nondominant hand.
7. Aspirate for blood return. If blood is aspirated, withdraw and discard needle. Apply gentle pressure as needed, and cover site with a bandage. Prepare a new injection and select a new site.
8. Inject medication slowly if no blood is aspirated and remove needle quickly at same angle as injection.

Deltoid Site

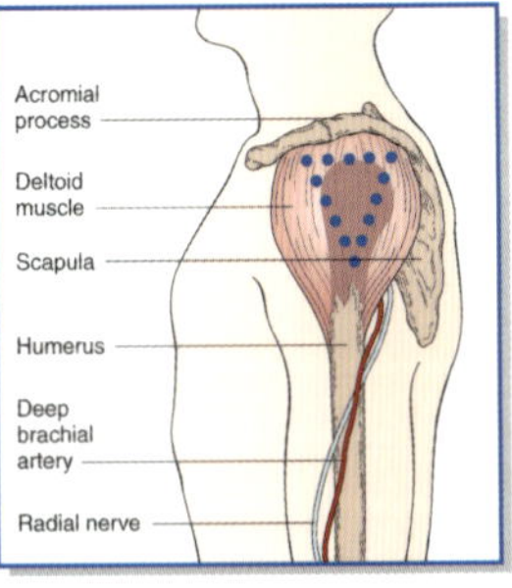

Ventrogluteal Site

Anterior superior iliac spine
Iliac crest
Gluteus medius
Greater trochanter

Vastus Lateralis Site

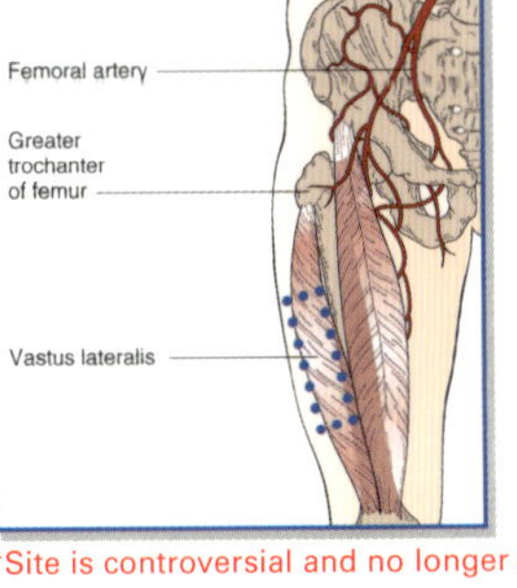

Dorsogluteal Site*

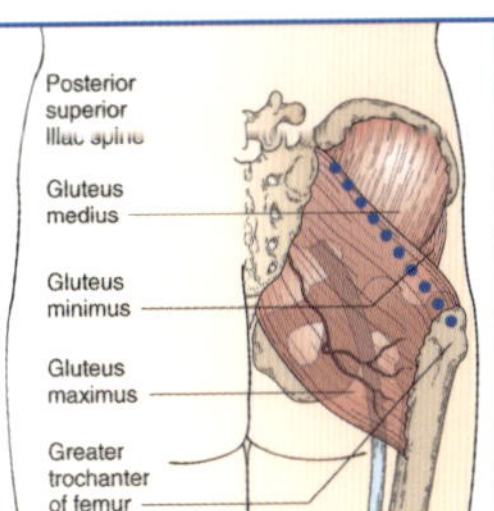

*Site is controversial and no longer recommended in some institutions.

Injections—Intramuscular Z-Track Method

1. Prepare injection. Draw up prescribed amount of medication and an additional 0.2–0.5 mL of air to create an air lock after injection.
2. Replace needle.
3. Don gloves.
4. Cleanse site with antiseptic, using moderate friction in a circular motion, moving outward from injection site. Avoid touching injection site once prepped.
5. Identify injection site (ventrogluteal or dorsogluteal preferred).
6. Pull skin taut from midline to one side, using nondominant hand.
7. Hold syringe so that air bubble floats to plunger, opposite the needle.
8. While maintaining skin retraction, insert needle at a 90° angle.
9. Aspirate for blood return. If blood aspirated, withdraw and discard needle, apply gentle pressure as needed, cover site with a bandage, and prepare a new injection for a new site.
10. Inject medication (including air bubble) slowly and smoothly. Hold needle in place for 10 sec.
11. Remove needle at same angle of injection while releasing skin.
12. Cover site with adhesive bandage if needed. ◎ Do not massage site after medication is injected.

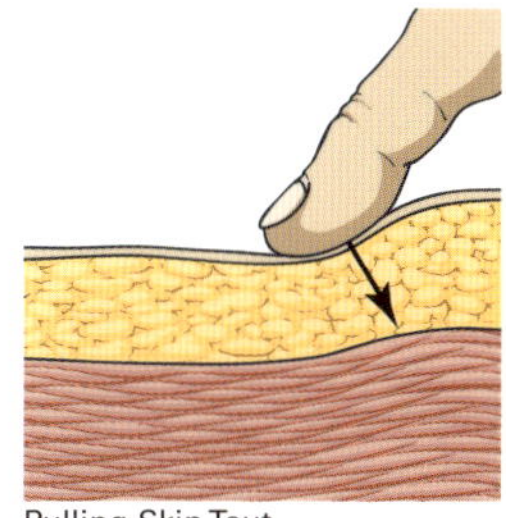

Pulling Skin Taut

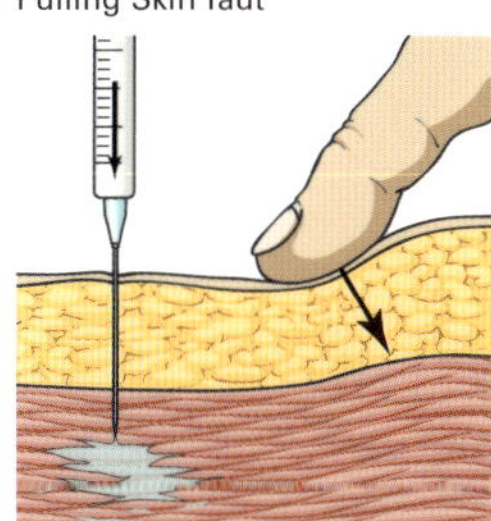

Inject

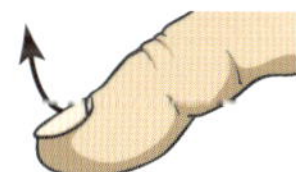

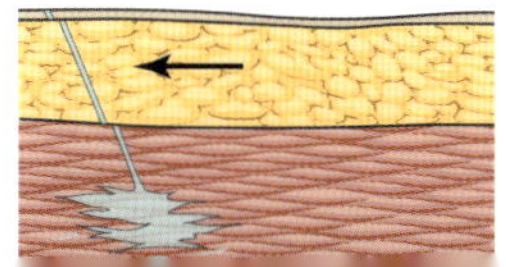

ANTICOAGULANT ALERT!

◎ **Heparin** should only be injected into the abdomen to decrease bleeding and bruising; **low molecular-weight heparin** should only be injected into the right or left sides of the abdomen to decrease pain and bruising.

◎ Draw up medication with additional 0.2 mL air to ensure all medication is injected and to create an air lock.

◎ Do not aspirate before injection or massage site after injection because it increases risk of bleeding or bruising.

INSULIN ALERT!

◎ Insulin syringes are measured in units and are NOT interchangeable with tuberculin (TB) syringes.

1. Position Pt according to injection site. If injecting heparin, use abdomen at a site farthest from previous injection, at least 2 in. from umbilicus. Rotate sites.
2. Don gloves.
3. Cleanse site with antiseptic using moderate friction in a circular motion, moving outward from injection site. Avoid touching injection site once prepared.
4. Pinch or spread skin. If less than 1 in. can be pinched between fingers, pinch skin and insert needle at a 45° angle. If more than 1 in. can be pinched, spread skin and insert needle at a 90° angle.
5. Insert needle with a quick, smooth motion.
6. Inject medication slowly. Aspirating for blood return before injection is not necessary, because inadvertent entry into a blood vessel is highly unlikely.
7. Remove needle quickly at same angle as injection.
8. Gently wipe site with an alcohol swab and cover with a bandage.
9. Avoid massaging site after injection unless specifically instructed. Rubbing may alter the rate of absorption.

Injections—Subcutaneous and Intradermal Sites

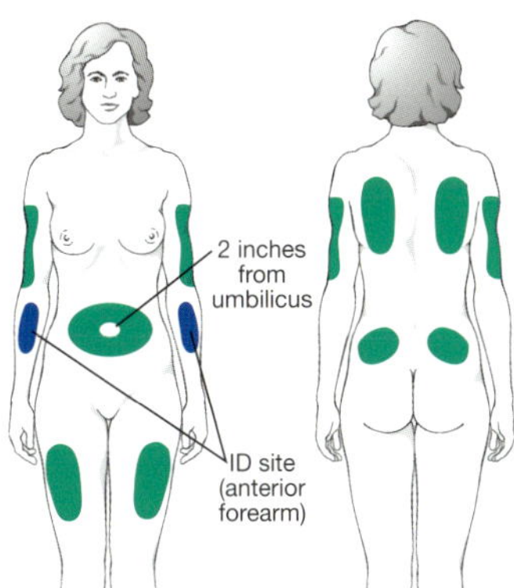

NCLEX Insulin—Mixing Technique

◎ Use only insulin syringes when mixing insulin.

◎ Do not dilute or mix with noninsulin medications.

1. Clean each vial seal with an alcohol swab.
2. Aspirate enough air into insulin syringe that is equal to volume of NPH to be withdrawn.
3. Maintain NPH vial in an upright position. Pressurize NPH vial, being careful not to contact solution. Remove syringe and set NPH vial aside.
4. Aspirate enough air into insulin syringe that is equal to volume of regular insulin to be withdrawn. Inject air into regular insulin vial, then withdraw exact amount of desired volume of regular insulin. Remove syringe and expel any air bubbles.
5. Insert syringe back into NPH vial (already pressurized), and withdraw exact amount of desired volume of NPH.

◎ Avoid pushing plunger and injecting regular insulin into NPH vial.

NCLEX Insulin—Types

Insulin Type	Onset	Peak	Duration
Rapid-Acting Insulin			
Insulin lispro (Humalog)	5 min	60–90 min	4–6 hr
Insulin aspart (Novolog)	10–20 min	1–3 hr	3–5 hr
Short-Acting Insulin			
Regular insulin (Humulin R) Only insulin that can be given IV.	Sub-Q route: 30–60 min IV route: 10–30 min	Sub-Q route: 2–4 hr IV route: 15–30 min	Sub-Q route: 5–7 hr IV route: 30–60 min
Concentrated insulin (Insulin U-500) Do not give by IV route.	30–60 min	2–3 hr	5–7 hr
Intermediate-Acting Insulin			
NPH (Humulin N, Novolin R)	1–2 hr	8–12 hr	18–24 hr
Long-Acting Insulin			
Insulin glargine (Lantus) Cannot be mixed with other insulins.	3–4 hr	None	24 hr
Insulin detemir (Levemir)	3–4 hr	3–14 hr	24 hr
Premixed Insulin			
NPH/regular (Humulin 50/50, Humulin 70/30; Novolin 70/30)	30 min	4–8 hr	24 hr
Aspart protamine/aspart (NovoLog Mix 70/30)	15 min	1–4 hr	24 hr
Lispro protamine/lispro (Humalog Mix 75/25)	15–30 min	2–8 hr	24 hr

Intravenous (IV)—Access, Infusion, Maintenance

Supplies

- Tourniquet
- Tape
- Warm pack
- Antiseptic swab
- Sterile dressing
- Non-latex gloves
- Appropriate-sized IV catheter

Access—Inserting a Peripheral IV or Saline Lock

◎ Inquire about Pt allergies, specifically to adhesives, iodine, or latex, and inquire about limb alert restrictions.

◎ Follow facility policy regarding the use of numbing creams and ID injection of local anesthetic for IV starts.

1. Apply tourniquet proximal to insertion site.
2. Palpate vein with fingertips. To further enhance dilation, gently tap vein, have Pt clinch fist repeatedly, or dangle arm below heart. Tip: Place a warm pack over insertion site or wrap thorax in warm blanket for 2–3 min before using tourniquet.
3. Cleanse site with antiseptic using moderate friction in a circular motion, moving outward from insertion site. Allow to air-dry.
4. Put on gloves. Avoid touching insertion site once prepared.
5. Inject numbing agent (if using). Discard needle in sharps container.
6. Apply traction. Stretch the skin in the opposite direction of catheter insertion.
7. Insert needle bevel side up at 15°–30°.
8. Observe for "flash back" (presence of blood) in flash chamber. Lower needle almost parallel to skin and advance 3–4 mm (ensures catheter is in vein).
9. Advance catheter to hub while maintaining skin traction.
10. Stabilize catheter and release tourniquet. Apply digital pressure just above end of catheter tip while gently stabilizing hub of catheter.
11. Remove needle, engage safety mechanism (if using a safety needle), and discard in sharps container.
12. Connect primed access apparatus:
    - **IV tubing:** Open clamp and observe for free flow of fluid (adjust rate).
    - **Saline lock:** Flush with NS to verify patency (engage slide clamp after flushing).

Infusion—Continuous

- Verify medication rights and triple-check order.
- Follow institution policy regarding use of infusion pumps.
- Document medication, infusion rate, date, and time.

As a Primary Line

1. Ensure compatibility if medication being added to primary bag.
2. Set infusion rate according to health-care provider orders.

As a Secondary Line (Through the Primary)

1. Ensure medication is compatible with primary IV solution.
2. Clean injection port with alcohol swab for 30 sec. Use injection port below primary line roller clamp; this allows for independent adjustment of flow rates without altering the other line.
3. Set secondary infusion rate according to health-care provider orders; both primary and secondary infusions run simultaneously at independent rates.

Infusion—Intermittent IV Piggyback (IVPB)

Refer to Medication—Administration

1. Verify medication rights, ensure IVPB bag is correctly labeled, confirm medication is compatible with primary IV solution, and ensure IVPB tubing is primed.
2. Follow institution policy regarding use of infusion pumps.
3. IVPB bag must be higher than primary IV bag. Hang primary bag from an extension hook so that it is lower than the IVPB bag.
4. Clean proximal injection port on primary line with alcohol swab for 30 sec.
5. Connect primed IVPB line to cleaned injection port.
6. Adjust IVPB roller clamp to desired rate.
7. Remove IVPB after infusion is complete and primary IV begins to infuse.
8. Confirm primary infusion rate is correct.

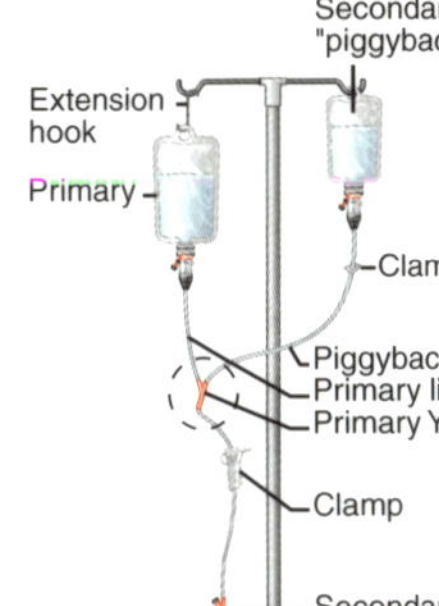

IVPB setup

Infusion—IV Push Medications

◎ Verify allergies, medication rights, and triple-check order. Use second nurse if required to verify and/or cosign any calculation.

◎ Ensure compatibility with IV solution.

- Use filter needle if drawing medication up from a glass ampule.
- Dilute medication (if needed) according to pharmacy policy.
- Document medication, dose, route, date, and time.

Through a Primary IV Line

1. Clean distal injection port with alcohol swab for 30 sec.
2. Inject medication over appropriate time interval.
3. If not compatible with IV solution, stop primary IV and flush line with 10 mL saline. Pinch line above injection port and inject medication.
4. Clear line of residual medication by flushing with 10 mL 0.9% saline solution (normal saline). Resume previous rate.

Through a Saline Lock

1. Clean injection port with alcohol swab for 30 sec.
2. Flush with 3–5 mL normal saline.
3. Inject medication over appropriate time interval.
4. Flush with 3–5 mL normal saline.
5. Discard syringe and/or needle in sharps container.

Maintenance—Flushing Peripheral and Central Lines

◎ Always verify heparin strength (10 or 100 units/mL)!

◎ Heparin flushes should never exceed 100 units/mL!

Device	Solution (per lumen)	Frequency
Peripheral Vascular Access Device (VAD)		
Peripheral IV line	3–5 mL NS (0.9% NaCl)	Every 12 hr and after each use
Midline catheter	5–10 mL NS followed with 1 mL heparin (10 units/mL)	Every 12 hr and after each use
Peripherally Inserted Central Catheters (PICCs)		
Groshong PICC	5–10 mL NS	Weekly and after each use
Per-Q-Cath (pediatric VAD)	3–5 mL NS followed with 1 mL heparin (10 units/mL)	Every 12 hr and after each use
Central Venous Catheters (CVC)		
Valve-tipped (no clamps)	5–10 mL NS	Weekly and after each use
Open-ended (clamps)	3–5 mL NS followed with 1 mL heparin (10 units/mL)	Every 12 hr and after each use
Implanted Port Catheters		
Groshong Port-A-Cath	5–10 mL NS followed with 1 mL heparin (100 units/mL)	Every 28 days and after each use

Routine Care of Peripheral and Central Lines

Clamps: Open-ended catheters—flush with heparin.
No Clamps: Valve-tip catheters do not have clamps—flush with NS using positive-pressure flush technique.
End-Caps: Change every 7 days or as needed.
Syringe Size: Use 10-mL syringe or greater—smaller syringes produce higher pressure, which can damage catheter.
Positive-Pressure Flush: Remove needle or needleless syringe while injecting last 0.5 mL of NS.

Troubleshooting IV Complications

Blood Backing Up Into IV Tubing

- Ensure IV bag has fluid and hang a new bag as needed. If bag is allowed to run dry, the tubing may fill with air; stop IV, attach a new bag, and reprime drip chamber. Insert a large syringe into a port distal to air and then clamp IV tubing distal to that port. Open roller clamp and aspirate air until tubing is reprimed.
- Ensure bag is hanging above both the level of the Pt's heart and the IV insertion site.
- Assess for unintentional, arterial cannulation; palpate for a pulse under insertion site and inspect for pulsation of blood in tubing. Discontinue IV and hold direct pressure for at least 5 min.

Decreased or No Infusion Rate

- Assess IV site for infiltration.
- Straighten extremity if IV insertion site is close to a joint.
- Maintain alignment of extremity with a padded arm board.
- Inspect entire length of tubing for kinks or holes.
- Inspect stopcocks and other flow-control devices.
- Ensure that burette (pediatrics) contains correct amount of fluid.
- Raise height of IV bag if not using an infusion pump.
- Flush with 3 mL of NS—if a significant amount of resistance is encountered, seek assistance per institutional policy. If assistance is unavailable, discontinue IV and start a new one, preferably on the opposite arm.

NCLEX Infiltration

- Assessment: Swelling, tenderness, decreased or no infusion rate, blanching of skin, site is cool to touch.
- Discontinue IV and restart in a new site. Apply warm compress to the affected area.

Leaking Fluid at IV Site

- Assess IV site for infiltration.
- Inspect connection between tubing and IV catheter.
- If all connections are patent, err on side of safety and assume that site is infiltrating or catheter is defective, even if IV is infusing freely. Call for an IV therapy consult.

NCLEX Pain at IV Site

- Assess IV site for infiltration, phlebitis, and irritation from tape.
- Ensure adequate stabilization of IV catheter.
- Straighten extremity if IV insertion site is close to a joint.
- Maintain alignment of extremity with a padded arm board.

discomfort.

Phlebitis

- Assessment: Classic sign is red line along course of vein. Other signs include redness, heat, swelling, and tenderness.
- Discontinue IV and restart in a new site. Apply warm compress to the affected area.

Intravenous Solution Types

IV solutions can be divided into two basic categories.

- **Crystalloids** contain water, dextrose, and/or electrolytes. These solutions are used to treat fluid and electrolyte imbalances.
- **Volume expanders** (often referred to as colloids or plasma expanders) have an increased osmotic pressure in comparison with crystalloids; they remain in the intravascular space longer. These solutions are used for volume expansion.

Crystalloids

Solution	Components	Indications
Saline solutions	Na and Cl (NS, 0.9% NaCl, sodium chloride).	Alkalosis, fluid loss, sodium depletion.
Dextrose solutions	Dextrose in water (D5W, D10W).	Caloric replacement, promote sodium diuresis, maintain water balance, prevent dehydration.
Dextrose and saline mixtures	Dextrose in saline (D5NS, D51/2NS, D10NS).	Promote diuresis, moderate fluid loss, prevent alkalosis, provide calories and sodium chloride.
Multielectrolyte solutions	Combination of Na, Cl, K, Ca, and lactate (LR).	Replace fluid lost from vomiting, GI suctioning, or dehydration.

Volume Expanders (Colloids)

The term *colloid* is often used to refer to all volume expanders.

- **Protein solutions:** Albumin, plasma, and commercial plasmas (e.g., Plasmanate).

- **Dextran:** Complex, synthetic sugar, metabolized slowly, does not stay in vascular space as long as a colloid.
- **Hetastarch:** Synthetic colloid that works similarly to Dextran.

Solution	Components	Indications
Albumin 5% and 25%	Human plasma protein.	• 5%—to expand volume and mobilize interstitial edema. • 25%—to treat hypoproteinemia.
Plasma	Contains human plasma proteins in NS (Plasmanate and plasma protein fraction).	• To increase serum colloid osmotic pressure.
Dextran 40 and 70	Synthetic colloid made of glucose polysaccharides.	• To expand volume. • To mobilize interstitial edema.
Hetastarch	Synthetic colloid made from corn (Hespan).	• To expand volume. • To mobilize interstitial edema.

Medication Errors

Prevention

- Always observe medication rights.
- Always triple-check all medications given.
- NCLEX Always confirm expiration date, strength, and route.
- NCLEX Always write out order; avoid using abbreviations or symbols.
- Always use commas for dosing units at or higher than 1,000.
- Always use adequate space among drug name, dose, and unit of measure.
- Always double-check dosage range with pharmacist.
- NCLEX Always have second nurse witness when mixing insulin and double-check dose and type of insulin you plan to administer.
- Always confirm dosage calculations and infusion pump programming.
- NCLEX Always clarify orders that are unclear or contain abbreviations.
- Always label all syringes and discard syringe immediately after use.
- If taking verbal order, ask prescriber to spell out drug name and dosage to avoid sound-alike confusion (e.g., hearing Cerebyx for Celebrex, or 50 for 15), and read back order to prescriber after you have written it in chart.
- Always document immediately after administering any medication.
- Always review each Pt's medications for the following:
  - Allergies, ADRs, and toxicity

- Overdose or subtherapeutic dose
- Medication duplication
- Potential drug or food interactions
- Weight changes requiring dosage adjustments
- Appropriate duration of therapy
- Adherence with prescribed medication therapy

- Never borrow medications from other Pts.
- Never administer medication drawn up by another person.
- Never document medication until after it has been administered.
- Never begin new medications before order has been received in pharmacy, because this circumvents built-in checks that can detect potential error.

Response

- Discontinue medication immediately.
- Assess for and treat symptoms of ADR.
- Ascertain whether Pt has known allergy to medication given.
- Notify health-care provider of medication error and any ADR.
- Document error (incident report) per institutional policy.
- Avoid using such phrases as "given in error."
- State facts only on MAR (medication, dose, time, route).
- In progress notes, document that health-care provider was notified.
- If there was any ADR, include intervention and outcome.

Do not document that an incident report was filed. NEVER record "medication error" on the MAR.

Pregnancy Risk Categories

- Category A: Adequate, well-controlled studies in pregnant women have not shown an increased risk of fetal abnormalities.
- Category B: (1) Animal studies show no adverse fetal effects, but there are no controlled human studies, or (2) animal studies show adverse fetal effect, but well-controlled human studies do not.
- Category C: (1) Animal studies show adverse fetal effect, but there are no controlled human studies, or (2) no animal or well-controlled human studies have been conducted.
- Category D: Well-controlled or observational human studies show positive evidence of human fetal risk. Maternal benefit may outweigh fetal risk in serious or life-threatening situations.
- Category X: Contraindicated. Well-controlled or observational human and/or animal studies show positive evidence of serious fetal abnormalities. Fetal risks far outweigh maternal benefit.

Basic Chemistry and Electrolytes

Reference ranges vary among facilities. Always check normal reference ranges from your facility's laboratory.

M, male; F, female.

Note: **Bold, red font (in parentheses)** indicates critical level.

Lab	Conventional	SI Units
Albumin	<1 yr: 2.9–5.5 g/dL 1–40 yr: 3.7–5.1 g/dL 41–60 yr: 3.4–4.8 g/dL 61–90 yr: 3.2–4.6 g/dL >90 yr: 2.9–4.5 g/dL	29–55 g/L 37–51 g/L 34–48 g/L 32–46 g/L 29–45 g/L
Aldolase (ALD)	0–2 yr: 3.4–11.8 units/L 2–16 yr: 1.2–8.8 units/L Adult: <7.4 units/L	3.4–11.8 units/L 1.2–8.8 units/L <7.4 units/L
Alkaline phosphatase	M: 35–142 units/L F: 25–125 units/L	35–142 units/L 25–125 units/L
Ammonia	M: 27–102 mcg/dL F: 19–87 mcg/dL	19–73 mcmol/L 1462 mcmol/L
Amylase	30–110 units/mL	30–110 units/mL
Anion gap	8–16 mEq/L	8–16 mmol/L
Aspartate aminotransferase (AST; formerly known as SGOT)	0–9 days: 47–150 units/L 10 days–23 mo: 9–80 units/L M: 2–59 yr: 15–40 units/L M: 60–90 yr: 19–48 units/L F: 2–59 yr: 13–35 units/L F: 60–90 yr: 9–36 units/L	47–150 units/L 9–80 units/L 15–40 units/L 19–48 units/L 13–35 units/L 9–36 units/L
Bilirubin, direct (conjugated)	<0.3 mg/dL	<5 mcmol/L
Bilirubin, indirect (unconjugated)	<1.1 mg/dL	<19 mcmol/L
Bilirubin, total **(>15 mg/dL)**	0–1 day: 1.4–8.7 mg/dL 1–2 days: 3.4–11.5 mg/dL 3–5 days: 1.5–12.0 mg/dL >1 mo: 0.3–1.2 mg/dL	24–149 mcmol/L 58–97 mcmol/L 26–205 mcmol/L 5–21 mcmol/L

Continued

Blood urea nitrogen (BUN) (>100 mg/dL) (nondialysis Pts)	0–3 yr: 5–17 mg/dL 4–13 yr: 7–17 mg/dL 14–90 yr: 8–21 mg/dL >90 yr: 10–31 mg/dL	1.8–6.0 mmol/L 2.5–6.0 mmol/L 2.9–7.5 mmol/L 3.6–11.1 mmol/L
Calcitonin	M: <19 pg/mL F: <14 pg/mL	<19 ng/L <14 ng/L
Calcium (Ca^{++}) (<7; >12 mg/dL)	3–12 yr: 8.8–10.8 mg/dL Adult: 8.2–10.2 mg/dL	2.20–2.70 mmol/L 2.05–2.55 mmol/L
Carbon dioxide (CO_2) (<15; >40 mmol/L)	<2 yr: 13–29 mEq/L >2 yr: 23–29 mEq/L	13–29 mmol/L 23–29 mmol/L
Chloride (Cl^-) (<80; >115 mEq/L)	0–1 mo: 98–113 mEq/L >1 mo: 97–107 mEq/L	98–113 mmol/L 97–107 mmol/L
Cholesterol	<20 yr: <170 mg/dL >20 yr: <200 mg/dL	<4.4 mmol/L <5.18 mmol/L
Cortisol	a.m.: 5–25 mcg/dL p.m.: 3–16 mcg/dL	138–690 nmol/L 83–442 nmol/L
Creatine kinase (CK)	M: 50–204 units/L F: 36–160 units/L	50–204 units/L 36–160 units/L
Creatinine (>7.4 mg/dL)	1–5 yr: 0.3–0.5 mg/dL 6–10 yr: 0.5–0.8 mg/dL M: >10 yr: 0.6–1.2 mg/dL F: >10 yr: 0.5–1.1 mg/dL	27–44 mcmol/L 44–71 mcmol/L 53–106 mcmol/L 44–97 mcmol/L
Ferritin	M: ≥16 yr: 20–250 ng/mL F: 16–39 yr: 10–20 ng/mL F: ≥40 yr: 12–263 ng/mL	20–250 mcg/L 10–20 mcg/L 12–263 mcg/L
Folate	>2.5 ng/mL	>5.7 nmol/L
Glucose (<40; >400 mg/dL)	1 day: 40–60 mg/dL 2 days–2 yr: 50–80 mg/dL Child: 60–100 mg/dL Adult: 65–99 mg/dL	2.2–3.3 mmol/L 2.8–4.4 mmol/L 3.3–5.6 mmol/L 3.6–5.5 mmol/L
HDL	Optimal: >60 mg/dL	0.9–1.56 mmol/L
Ionized calcium (<3.2; >6.2 mg/dL)	4.6–5.08 mg/dL	1.12–1.32 mmol/L
Iron (Fe) (>400 mcg/dL)	M: 65–175 mcg/dL F: 50–170 mcg/dL	11.6–31.3 mcmol/L 9–30.4 mcmol/L
Iron binding capacity, total (TIBC)	250–350 mcg/dL	45–63 mcmol/L

Continued

Lab	Conventional	SI Units
K^+ (Potassium) (<2.5; >6.5)	Child: 3.4–4.7 mEq/L Adult: 3.5–5.0 mEq/L	3.4–4.7 mmol/L 3.5–5.0 mmol/L
Lactate dehydrogenase (LDH)	90–156 units/L	90–156 units/L
Lactic acid (≥31 mg/dL)	3–23 mg/dL	0.3–2.6 mmol/L
Lipase	3–73 units/L	3–73 units/L
Low-density lipoprotein (LDL)	Optimal: <100 mg/dL	<2.59 mmol/L
Magnesium (Mg^{++}) (<1.2; >4.9 mg/dL)	Child:1.7–2.1 mg/dL Adult: 1.6–2.6 mg/dL	0.70–0.86 mmol/L 0.66–1.07 mmol/L
Mg^{++} (magnesium) (<1.2; >4.9 mg/dL)	Child: 1.7–2.1 mg/dL Adult: 1.6–2.6 mg/dL	0.70–0.86 mmol/L 0.66–1.07 mmol/L
Na^+ (sodium) (<120; >160 mmol/L)	0–1 yr: 133–144 mEq/L >1 yr: 135–145 mEq/L	133–144 mmol/L 135–145 mmol/L
Osmolality (<265; >320 mOsm/kg)	275–295 mOsm/kg	275–295 mmol/kg
Phosphorus (<1 mg/dL)	2.5–4.5 mg/dL	0.8–1.4 mmol/L
Potassium (K^+) (<2.5; >6.5 mmol/L)	Child: 3.4–4.7 mEq/L Adult: 3.5–5.0 mEq/L	3.4–4.7 mmol/L 3.5–5.0 mmol/L
Prealbumin	12–42 mg/dL	120–420 mg/L
Protein, total	6–8 g/dL	60–80 g/L
Prostate-specific antigen (PSA)	<4 ng/mL	<4 mcg/L
Pyruvate kinase	9–22 international units/g hemoglobin	9–22 international units/g hemoglobin
Sodium (Na^+) (<120; >160 mmol/L)	0–1 yr: 133–144 mEq/L >1 yr: 135–145 mEq/L	133–144 mmol/L 135–145 mmol/L
Thyroglobulin	0–50 ng/mL	0–50 mcg/L
Thyroid-stimulating hormone (TSH)	0.4–4.2 microinternational units/mL	0.4–4.2 microinternational units/mL
Thyroxine (T_4) free	0.8–1.5 ng/dL	10–19 pmol/L
Thyroxine (T_4) total (<2 mcg/dL; >20 mcg/dL)	M: 4.6–10.5 mcg/dL F: 5.5–11 mcg/dL Gravid: 5.5–16 mcg/dL	59–135 nmol/L 71–142 nmol/L 71–155 nmol/L

Continued

Lab	Conventional	SI Units
Triglycerides	<150 mg/dL	<1.7 mmol/L
Tri-iodothyronine (T_3) free	260–480 pg/dL Gravid: 196–338 pg/dL	4–7.4 pmol/L 3–5.2 pmol/L
Tri-iodothyronine (T_3) total	70–204 ng/dL Gravid: 116–247 ng/dL	1.08–3.14 nmol/L 1.79–3.8 nmol/L
Urea nitrogen (>100 mg/dL)	Child: 7–17 mg/dL Adult: 8–21 mg/dL	2.5–6.0 mmol/L 2.9–7.5 mmol/L
Uric acid	M: 4.4–7.6 mg/dL F: 2.3–6.6 mg/dL	0.26–0.45 mmol/L 0.14–0.39 mmol/L

Blood Gas Analysis

Arterial Blood Gas

Lab	Conventional	SI Units
pH (<7.20; >7.60)	7.35–7.45	7.35–7.45
PO_2 (<45 mm Hg)	80–95 mm Hg	10.6–12.6 kPa
PCO_2 (<20; >67 mmHg)	35–45 mm Hg	4.66–5.98 kPa
HCO_3 (<10; >40 mmol/L)	18–23 mEq/L	18–23 mmol/L
Base excess	(−2)–(+3) mEq/L	(−2)–(+3) mmol/L
CO_2	22–29 mEq/L	22–29 mmol/L
O_2 Saturation	95%–100%	95%–100%

Venous Blood Gas

Lab	Conventional	SI Units
pH	7.32–7.43	7.32–7.43
PO_2	20–49 mm Hg	2.6–6.5 kPa
PCO_2	41–51 mm Hg	5.4–6.8 kPa
HCO_3	24–28 mEq/L	24–28 mmol/L
CO_2	25–30 mEq/L	25–30 mmol/L
O_2 Saturation	70%–75%	70%–75%

Acid–Base Imbalance

Imbalance	pH	PCO_2	PO_2	HCO_3	Compensation
Respiratory Acidosis					Kidneys conserve HCO_3; eliminate H^+ to ↑ pH
Uncompensated	↓	↑	Normal	Normal	
Compensated	Normal	↑	↑	↑	
Respiratory Alkalosis					Kidneys eliminate HCO_3; conserve H^+ to ↓ pH
Uncompensated	↑	↓	Normal	Normal	
Compensated	Normal	↓	↓	↓	
Metabolic Acidosis					Hyperventilation to blow off excess CO_2 and conserve HCO_3
Uncompensated	↓	Normal	↓	↓	
Compensated	Normal	↓	↓	↓	
Metabolic Alkalosis					Hypoventilation to ↑ CO_2 Kidneys keep H^+ and excrete HCO_3
Uncompensated	↑	Normal	↑	↑	
Compensated	Normal	↑	↑	↑	

NCLEX Common Causes of Acid–Base Imbalance

Respiratory acidosis	Asphyxia, respiratory and CNS depression.
Respiratory alkalosis	Hyperventilation, anxiety, diabetic ketoacidosis.
Metabolic acidosis	Diarrhea, renal failure, salicylate (aspirin) overdose.
Metabolic alkalosis	Hypercalcemia, alkaline (antacid) overdose.

Cardiac Markers

Lab	Conventional	SI Units
CK (total)	M: 50–204 units/L F: 36–160 units/L	50–204 units/L 36–160 units/L
CK–MB	0–3 ng/mL	0–3 ng/mL
LDH	90–156 units/L	90–156 units/L
Myoglobin	5–70 mcg/L	5–70 mcg/L
Troponin-I (>0.5 ng/mL)	<0.35 ng/mL	<0.35 ng/mL
Troponin-T	<0.20 mcg/mL	<0.20 mcg/mL

Progression of Cardiac Markers

Lab	Onset	Peak	Duration
AST (SGOT)	6–8 hr	12–48 hr	3–4 days
CK (total)	4–6 hr	24 hr	2–3 days
CK-MB	4–6 hr	15–20 hr	2–3 days
LDH	12 hr	24–48 hr	10–14 days
Myoglobin	1–3 hr	4–12 hr	1 day
Troponin-I	2–6 hr	15–20 hr	5–7 days
Troponin-T	3–5 hr	24 hr	10–15 days

Cerebrospinal Fluid (CSF)

Lab (Lumbar Puncture)	Conventional	SI Units
Color	Crystal clear	Crystal clear
Protein	15–45 mg/dL	150–450 mg/L
Glucose	40–70 mg/dL	2.2–3.9 mmol/L
Lactic acid	<25.2 mg/dL	<2.8 mmol/L
Myelin basic protein	<4 ng/mL	<4 mcg/L
Oligoclonal bands	Absent	Absent
Immunoglobulin G	<3.4 mg/dL	<34 mg/L
Gram stain	Negative	Negative

Continued

Lab (Lumbar Puncture)	Conventional	SI Units
India ink	Negative	Negative
Culture	No growth	No growth
RBC count	Zero	Zero
WBC count	0–5/mL	0–5 × 10^6/L

Coagulation

Lab	Conventional	SI Units
Activated coagulation time (ACT)	90–130 sec	90–130 sec
Activated partial thromboplastin time (aPTT) (>70 sec)	25–39 sec	25–39 sec
Bleeding time (>14 min)	2–7 min	2–7 min
Fibrinogen (<80 mg/dL)	200–400 mg/dL	2–4 g/L
International normalized ratio (INR) (>5)	Normal: <2 Target therapeutic: 2–3	<2 2–3
Plasminogen	80%–120% of normal	80%–120% of normal
Platelets (<20,000; >1,000,000)	150,000–450,000/mm^3	150–450 × 10^9/L
Prothrombin time (PT) (>27 sec)	10–13 sec	10–13 sec
Thrombin time	11–15 sec	11–15 sec

Disseminated Intravascular Coagulopathy Panel

Lab	Conventional	SI Units
aPTT (activated) (>70 sec)	25–39 sec	25–39 sec
PT (>27 sec)	10–13 sec	10–13 sec
Fibrinogen (<80 mg/dL)	200–400 mg/dL	2–4 g/L
Thrombin time	11–15 sec	11–15 sec
D-Dimer	<300 ng/mL	<300 ng/mL

Hematology (CBC With Differential)

Lab	Conventional	SI Units
Blood volume	8.5%–9.0% of body weight in kg	80–85 mL/kg
Red blood cell (RBC)	M: 4.71–5.14 × 10^6 cells/mm^3 F: 4.20–4.87 × 10^6 cells/mm^3	4.71–5.14 × 10^{12} cells/L 4.20–4.87 × 10^{12} cells/L
Hemoglobin (Hgb) **(<6; >18 g/dL)**	M: 13.2–17.3 g/dL F: 11.7–15.5 g/dL	132–173 mmol/L 117–155 mmol/L
Hematocrit (Hct) **(<18; >54%)**	M: 43%–49% F: 38%–44%	0.43%–0.49% 0.38%–0.44%
Leukocytes (WBC) **(<2500; >30,000/mm^3)**	4.5–11 × 10^3/mm^3	4.5–11 × 10^9/L
• Neutrophils **• Bands** **• Segments**	59% 3.0% 56%	0.59 0.03 0.56
• Lymphocytes	34%	0.34
• Monocytes	4.0%	0.04
• Eosinophils	2.7%	0.027
• Basophils	0.5%	0.005
Platelets **(<20,000; >1,000,000)**	150,000–450,000/mm^3	150–450 × 10^9/L
Erythrocyte sedimentation rate (ESR)	M: 0–49 yr: 0–15 mm/hr M: >49 yr: 0–20 mm/hr F: 0–49 yr: 0–25 mm/hr F: >49 yr: 0–30 mm/hr	0–15 mm/hr 0–20 mm/hr 0–25 mm/hr 0–30 mm/hr

Medication Levels (Therapeutic)

Medication	Conventional	Critical/Toxic	SI Units
Acetaminophen	10–30 mcg/mL	After 4 hr: >150 After 12 hr: >50	66–199 mcmol/L
Amiodarone	0.5–2.0 mg/L	>2	
Carbamazepine	4–12 mcg/mL	>12	17–51 mcmol/L
Digoxin	0.5–2.0 ng/mL	>2.5	0.6–2.6 nmol/L
Lidocaine	1.5–5.0 mcg/mL	>6	6.4–21.4 mcmol/L
Lithium	0.6–1.4 mEq/L	>1.5	0.6–1.4 mEq/L

Continued

Medication	Conventional	Critical/Toxic	SI Units
Nitroprusside	<10 mg/dL	>10	
Phenobarbital	15–40 mcg/mL	>40	65–172 mcmol/L
Phenytoin	10–20 mcg/mL	>20	40–79 mcmol/L
Procainamide	4–10 mcg/mL	>12	17–42 mcmol/L
Propranolol	50–100 ng/mL	>150	
Quinidine	2–5 mcg/mL	>8	6–15 mcmol/L
Salicylate	15–20 mg/dL	>30	1.1–1.4 mmol/L
Theophylline	10–20 mcg/mL	>20	

Antibiotic Levels (Peak and Trough)

Antibiotic	Peak	Critical	Trough	Critical
Amikacin	C: 20–30 mcg/mL SI: 34–51 mcmol/L	>30 >51	1–8 mcg/mL 2–14 mcmol/L	>8 >14
Gentamicin	C: 6–10 mcg/mL SI: 12–21 mcmol/L	>12 >25	0.5–1.5 mcg/mL 1–3 mcmol/L	>2 >3
Tobramycin	C: 6–10 mcg/mL SI: 12–21 mcmol/L	>12 >26	0.5–1.5 mcg/mL 1–3 mcmol/L	>2 >3
Vancomycin	C: 30–40 mcg/mL SI: 21–28 mcmol/L	>80 >55	5–10 mcg/mL 3–7 mcmol/L	>20 >14

C, conventional; SI, SI units.

Urinalysis

Lab	Conventional
Appearance	Clear
Color	Yellow (straw)
pH	5.0–9.0
Protein	<20 mg/dL
Glucose	Negative
Ketones	Negative
Hemoglobin	Negative
Bilirubin	Negative

Urobilinogen	≤1 mg/dL
Nitrite	Negative
Leukocyte esterase	Negative
Specific gravity	1.001–1.029
Osmolality	250–900 mOsm/kg
RBC	<5/hpf
WBC	<5/hpf
Renal cells	None seen
Transitional cells	None seen
Squamous cells	Rare; usually not significant
Casts	Rare hyaline; otherwise, none seen

Basic ECG Interpretation

Cardiac Anatomy and Conduction

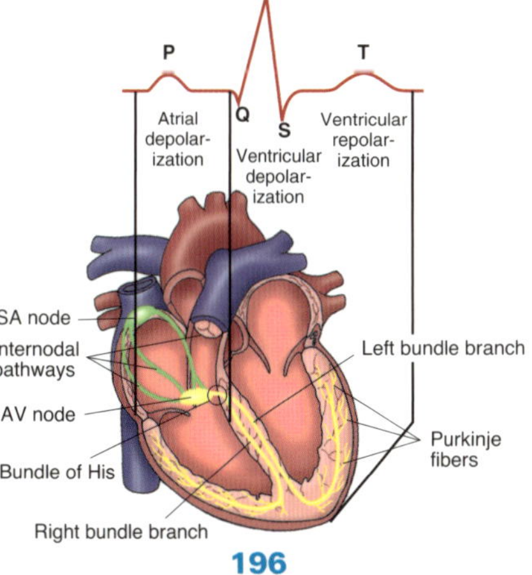

ECG Components

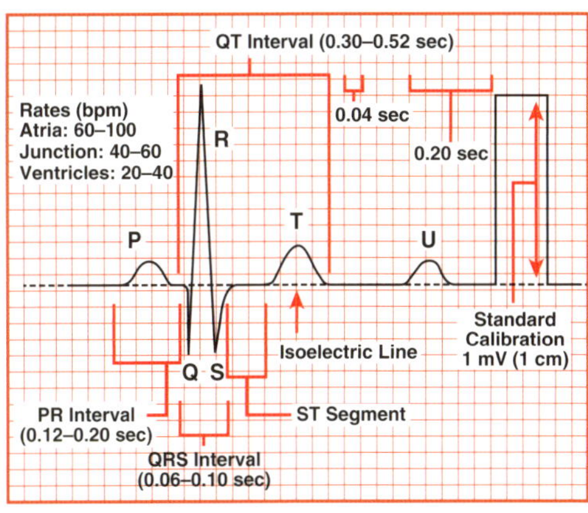

ECG Parameters

Normal sinus rhythm	60–100 bpm
Sinus bradycardia	<60 bpm
Sinus tachycardia	>100 bpm
Supraventricular tachycardia	>150 bpm
QRS complex	0.06–0.10 sec
PR interval	0.12–0.20 sec
Atrial rate, inherent	60–100 bpm
Junctional rate, inherent	40–60 bpm
Ventricular rate, inherent	20–40 bpm

ECG Systematic Assessment

Rate	Is it normal (60–100), fast (>100), or slow (< 60)?
Rhythm	Is it regular, irregular?
P waves	Are they present? Are they 1:1 with the QRS?
PR interval	Is it normal (0.12–0.2 sec)? Does it remain consistent?
QRS complex	Is it normal (0.06–0.10 sec), or is it wide (>0.10 sec)?
Extra	Are there any extra or abnormal complexes?

Analyzing the PR Interval (PRI)

Finding	Conclusion
PRI is consistent, and normal, between 0.12 and 0.20 sec (3–5 small boxes).	Normal PRI.
PRI is <0.12 sec (3 small boxes).	Junctional rhythm.
PRI is >0.20 sec (5 small boxes), it remains consistent in length from PRI to PRI.	1° AV block.
Progressive lengthening of PRI until QRS is dropped.	2° AV block type I (Mobitz I or Wenckebach).
Consistent PRI; however, there are additional P waves that do not precede a QRS complex.	2° AV block type II (Mobitz II).
PRI is not consistent, nor is there any correlation between P wave and QRS.	3° AV block (complete heart block).

Analyzing the QRS

Finding	Conclusion
QRS ≤0.10 sec.	Normal.
QRS >0.10 sec, "wide and bizarre."	Ventricular ectopy.
QRS >0.10 sec (2.5 small boxes), with notched or "rabbit ears" appearance.	BBB (see differentiating RBBB from LBBB).
QRS proceeded by 1–2 very narrow "spikes."	Pacemaker.

Lead Placement—Standard Three- and Five-Wire

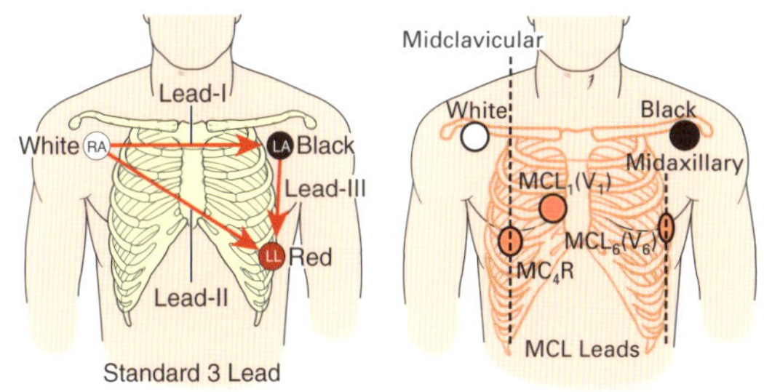

12-Lead ECG

12-Lead Placement—Chest and Limb Leads

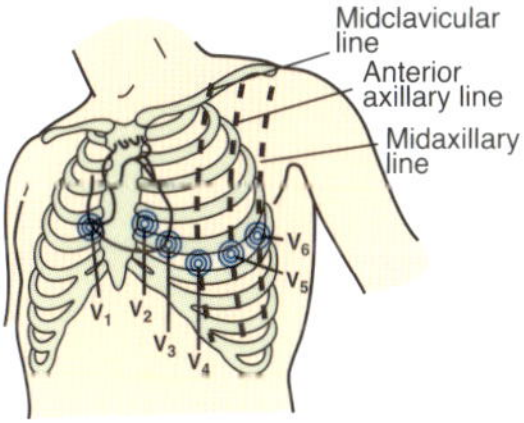

Midclavicular line
Anterior axillary line
Midaxillary line
V_1 V_2 V_3 V_4 V_5 V_6

- **V_1**: 4th ICS, right sternal border
- **V_2**: 4th ICS, left sternal border
- **V_3**: midway between V_2 and V_4
- **V_4**: 5th ICS, midclavicular line
- **V_5**: 5th ICS, midway between V_4 and V_6
- **V_6**: 5th ICS, midaxillary line

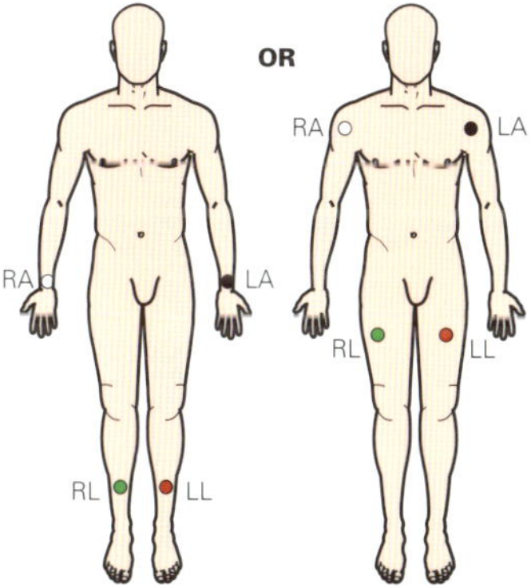

RA LA RL LL

OR

RA LA RL LL

Differentiating RBBB From LBBB

LBBB	RBBB
QRS: >0.10 sec.	**QRS**: >0.10 sec.
V_1, V_2: Predominantly negative (QS in V_1).	**V_1, V_2**: Predominantly positive, rSR′ or rR′ (rabbit ears).
I, V_5, V_6: Blunted, upright QRS with T wave inversion.	**I, V_5, V_6**: Slurred S wave.

Differentiating Wide-Complex Tachycardia

SVT With Aberrancy	Ventricular Tachycardia
I, aVL: Positive **V_1**: Triphasic Associated P waves	**I, aVL**: Negative **V_1**: Biphasic or positive **aVR**: Positive Concordance in V_1–V_6 (all negative or all positive) Fusion or capture beats

Localizing Ischemia on 12-Lead

Assess Quality of 12-Lead Tracing

- Lead aVR should have a predominantly negative deflection.
- Confirm 1 mV (two large boxes) of standard calibration.

Look for Lead Changes Suggestive of an MI*

- **LBBB (new)**: *Diagnosis of AMI is confounded by LBBB.
- **QRS**: >0.10 sec.
- **V_1, V_2**: Predominantly negative (QS in V_1).
- **T-wave inversion** (ischemia): Should appear symmetrical. T-wave inversion in I, V_5, V_6 is suggestive of LBBB.
- **ST elevation** (injury): 1 mm or more of ST elevation in two or more contiguous leads confirms MI. Elevation is usually associated with reciprocal ST depression in other leads.
- **Significant Q waves** (infarct): Suggestive of MI. A large Q wave is normal in aVR (not used in diagnosing AMI). Small Q waves (<0.4 sec) can be normal in leads I, aVL, V_5, V_6.
- **ST depression** (consistent with NSTEMI): May be present in V_1–V_4 without reciprocal ST elevation (posterior MI).

Patterns of Acute MI

ST Elevation Pattern	Area of MI	Related Findings
II, III, and aVF	Inferior	↓ BP, use NTG/MS with caution.
I, aVL, V_5, V_6	Lateral	LV dysfunction, AV blocks.
V_1, V_2	Septal	BBBs common.
V_3, V_4	Anterior	CHF, 3° HB, BBBs common.
V_4R–V_6R	RV	↓ BP, A-fib/flutter, PACs, AV blocks.
V_1–V_4 (ST depression)	Posterior	LV dysfunction.

Reciprocal Lead Changes of Acute MI

Leads With ST Elevation	Reciprocal ST Depression
II, III, aVF	I, aVL, V_3, V_4
I, aVL, V_5, V_6	II, III, aVF
V_3, V_4	II, III, aVF
No ST elevation (NSTEMI?)	V_1–V_4 (suspect posterior MI)

Sample ECG Rhythms

Asystole

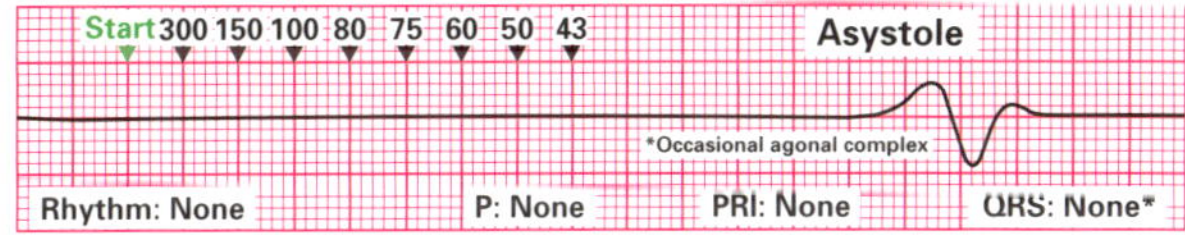

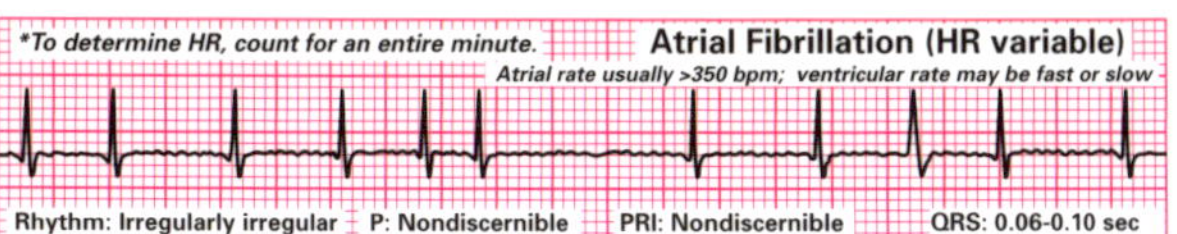

Atrial Flutter (A-Flutter)

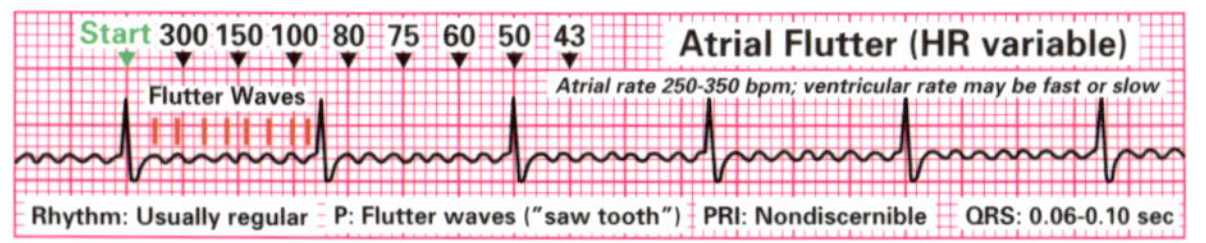

Atrioventricular (AV) Block—First Degree

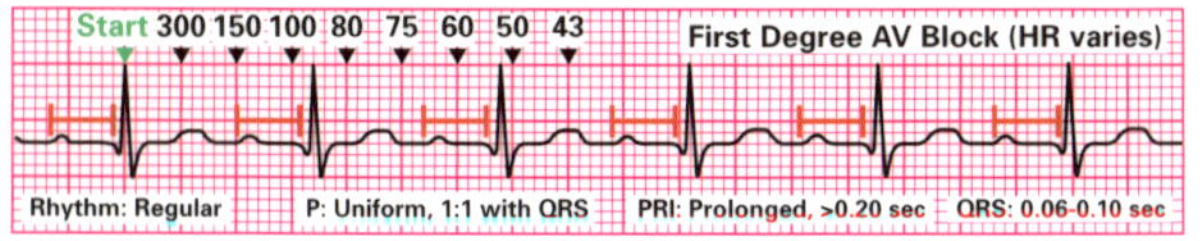

Atrioventricular (AV) Block—Second Degree Type I

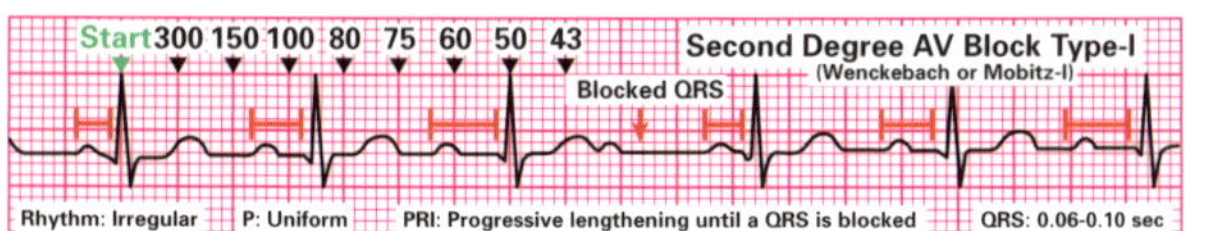

Atrioventricular (AV) Block—Second Degree Type II

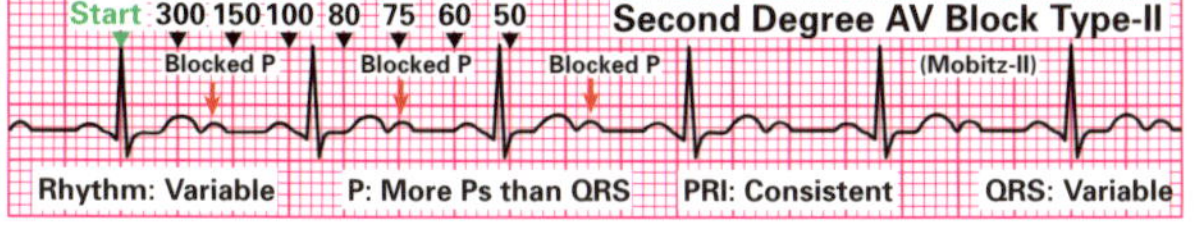

Atrioventricular (AV) Block—Third Degree

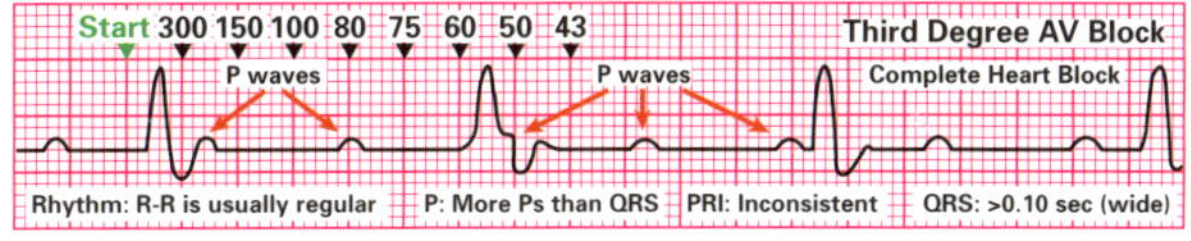

Junctional Rhythm

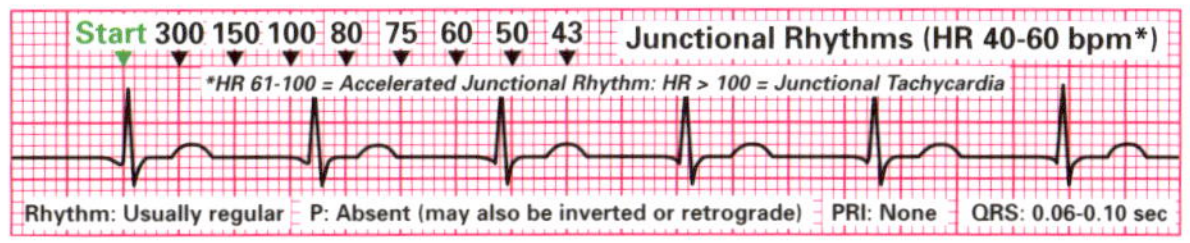

Pacemaker Rhythm

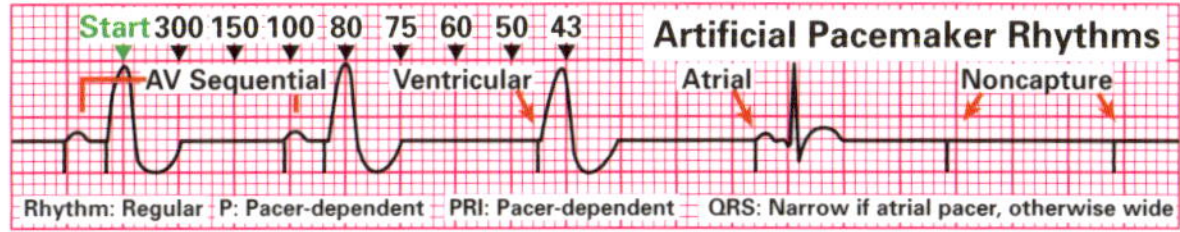

Premature Atrial/Junctional Complex (PAC/PJC)

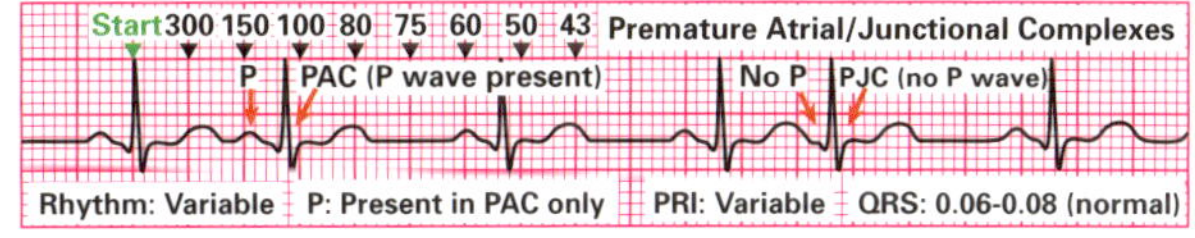

Premature Ventricular Complex (PVC)

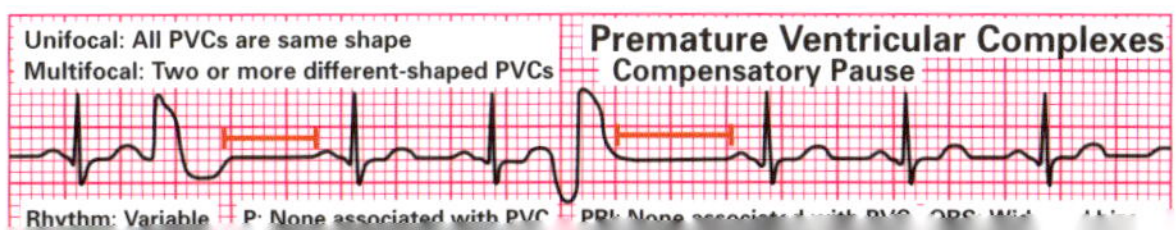

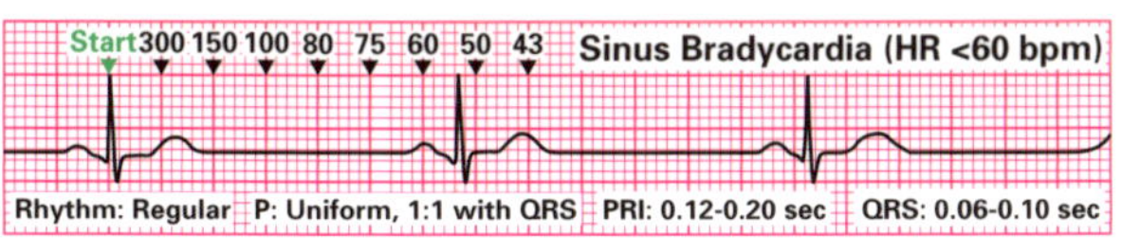

Sinus Rhythm (SR; also NSR = normal sinus rhythm)

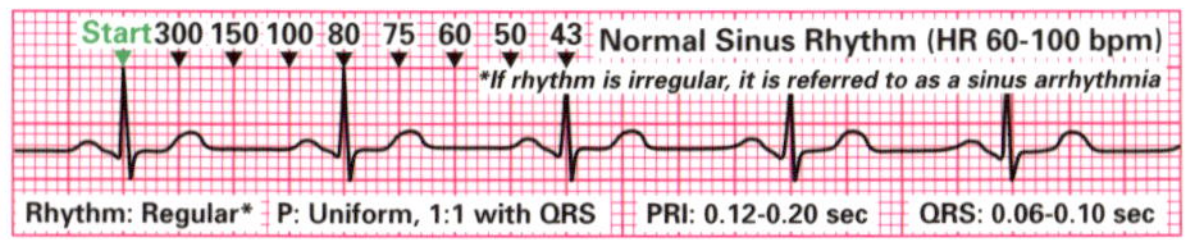

Sinus Tachycardia (ST)

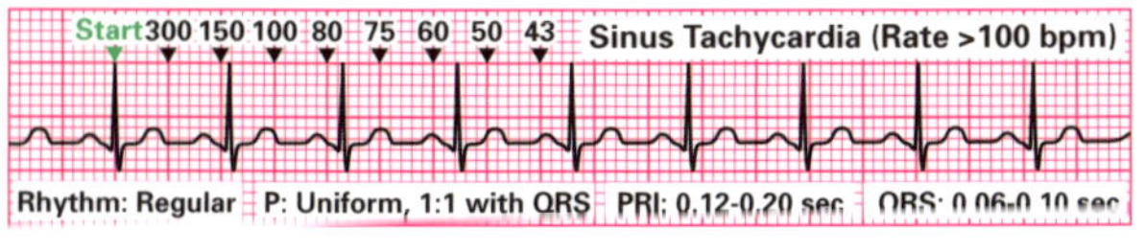

Torsade de Pointes (twisting of points)

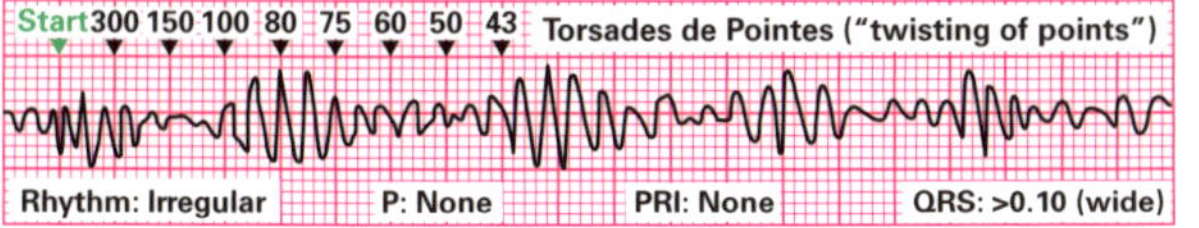

Ventricular Fibrillation (coarse V-Fib)

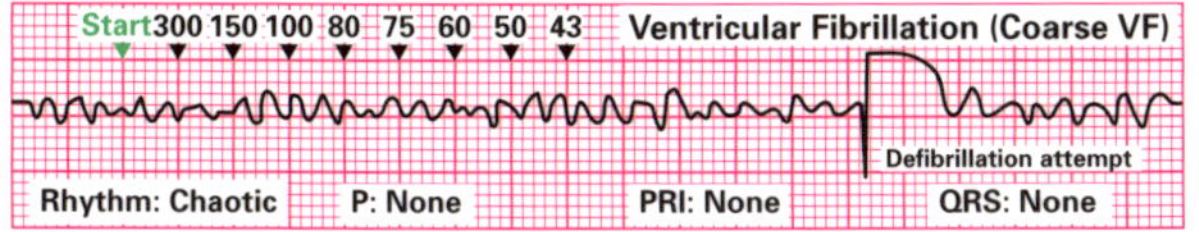

Ventricular Fibrillation (fine V-Fib)

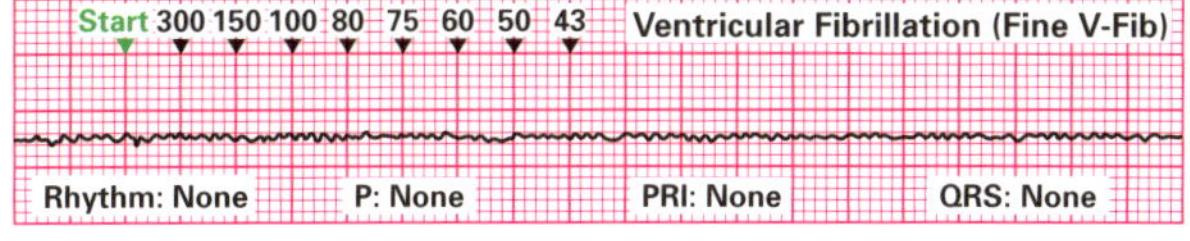

Ventricular Tachycardia (VT)—Monomorphic

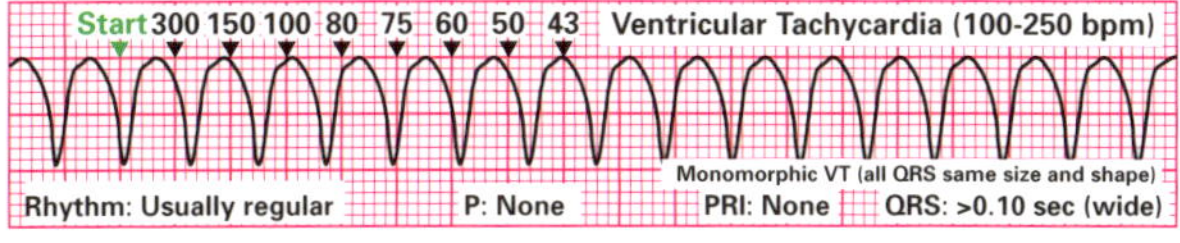

Ventricular Tachycardia (VT)—Polymorphic

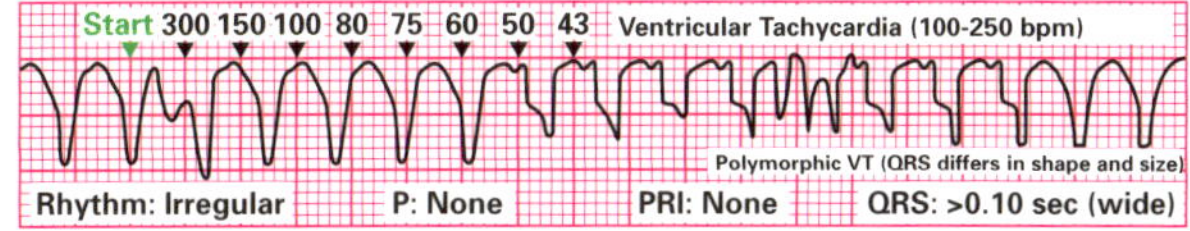

Wolff-Parkinson White (WPW)

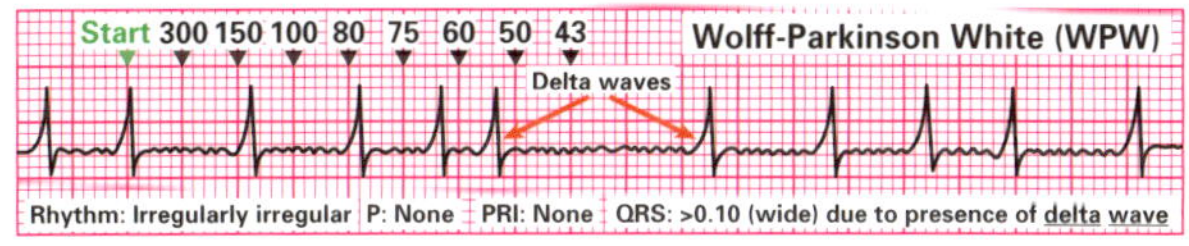

WPW is an abnormal accessory pathway that bypasses the normal route through the AV node. This prematurely depolarizes a portion of the ventricles and causes a delta wave (slurring of the initial portion of the QRS). PRI is shortened (nondiscernible in A-fib), and the QRS is widened >0.10 sec.

Alzheimer's Disease (AD)

Definition: This disabling degenerative disease of the nervous system is characterized by dementia and failure of memory for recent events, followed by total incapacitation and eventually death.

Clinical Findings:

Stage I: Loss of recent memory, irritability, loss of interest in life, and decline of abstract thinking and problem-solving ability.

Stage II: (Most common stage when disease is diagnosed) profound memory deficits, inability to concentrate or manage business or personal affairs.

Stage III: Aphasia, inability to recognize or use objects, involuntary emotional outbursts, and incontinence.

Stage IV: Nonverbal status and complete withdrawal; loss of appetite leading to emaciation; cessation of all bodily functions, and death ensuing quickly.

Nursing Focus

- Monitor vital signs and LOC, and implement collaborative care as ordered.
- Keep requests simple and avoid confrontation.
- Maintain a consistent environment and frequently reorient Pt.

Reinforce Patient Teaching

- Provide Pt and family with literature on AD.
- Advise family that, as AD progresses, so does need for supervision of ADLs such as cooking and bathing.
- Advise family to lock windows and doors to prevent wandering.
- Explain that Pt should wear an ID bracelet in case he or she becomes lost.
- Explain actions, dosages, side effects, and adverse reactions of meds.

Asthma

Definition: Often referred to as *reactive airway disease* (RAD), asthma is an intermittent, reversible, obstructive lung disease characterized by bronchospasm and hyperreactivity to a multitude of triggering agents (allergens/antigens/irritants).

Clinical Findings: Difficulty breathing, wheezing, cough (either dry or productive of thick, white sputum), chest tightness, anxiety, prolonged expiratory phase, and use of accessory muscles.

Nursing Focus

- During an attack, assess and maintain ABCs, notify RT/MD, and implement collaborative care, such as meds and IV fluid, as ordered.
- Stay with Pt and offer emotional support.
- Monitor vital signs, and document response to prescribed therapies.

NCLEX Reinforce Patient Teaching

- Provide Pt and family with literature on asthma.
- Explain actions, dosages, side effects, and adverse reactions of meds.
- Provide instructions on proper use of metered-dose inhalers.
- Provide instructions on proper use of peak-flow meter.
- Provide instructions on implementing an asthma management plan.
- Teach Pt and family about kinds of triggering agents that can precipitate an attack and how to minimize risk of exposure.
- Instruct Pt to seek immediate medical attention if symptoms are not relieved with prescribed meds.

Cancer: General Overview

Definition: Malignant neoplasia is marked by uncontrolled growth of cells, often with invasion of healthy tissues locally or throughout the body (metastasis).

Clinical Findings: Vary with different types of cancer.

Types of Treatments

Surgery: Removing cancerous tissue surgically or by means of cryosurgery (technique for freezing and destroying abnormal cells).

Chemotherapy: Treatment of cancer with drugs ("anticancer" drugs) that destroy cancer cells or stop them from growing or multiplying. Because some drugs work better together than alone, two or more drugs are often given concurrently (combination therapy).

Radiation Therapy: Ionizing radiation (x-rays, gamma rays, or radioactive implants) depositing energy that injures or destroys cells in target tissue by damaging their genetic material and making continued growth impossible.

Palliative and Hospice Care: Care focused solely on minimizing pain and suffering when cure is not an option.

Nursing Focus

- **Nausea and Vomiting**: Administer antiemetics as needed and before chemotherapy is initiated. Withhold foods and fluids 4–6 hr before chemotherapy. Provide small portions of bland foods after each treatment.
- **Diarrhea**: Administer antidiarrheals. Monitor electrolytes. Give clear liquids as tolerated. Maintain good perineal care.
- **Stomatitis**: Avoid commercial mouthwash containing alcohol. Encourage good oral hygiene. Help Pt rinse with viscous lidocaine before eating to reduce discomfort and again after meals. Apply water-soluble lubricant to cracked lips. Popsicles provide a good source of moisture.
- **Itching**: Keep Pt's skin free of foreign substances. Avoid soap: wash with plain water and pat dry. Use cornstarch or olive oil to relieve itching, and avoid talcum powder and powder with zinc oxide.

- Provide Pt and family with literature for specific type of cancer.
- Prepare Pt and family for what to expect with chemotherapy and radiation therapy.
- If surgery is to be performed, provide preoperative teaching to prepare Pt and family for procedure and postoperative care. Provide discharge instructions.
- Explain actions, dosages, side effects, and adverse reactions of meds.

Tumor Facts

- **Benign Tumors:** Noncancerous. They can often be removed, and in most cases, do not come back. Cells from benign tumors do not spread to other parts of the body. Most importantly, benign tumors are rarely a threat to life.
- **Malignant Tumors:** Cancerous. Cells in these tumors are abnormal and divide without control or order. They can invade and damage nearby tissues and organs.
- **Metastasis:** Process by which cancer cells break away from a malignant tumor, enter bloodstream or lymphatic system, and spread from original cancer site to form new tumors in other organs.

TNM Staging of Cancer

T: Tumor Size	N: Nodes Involved	M: Metastasis
T1 . . . . .Small	N0 . . . . . .No involvement	M0 . . . . .None
T2 or T3 . . .Medium	N1–N3 . . . . .Moderate	M1 . . . . . .Metastasis
T4 . . . . .Large	N4 . . . . .Extensive	

ABCDs of Melanoma

Asymmetry	Border	Color	Diameter
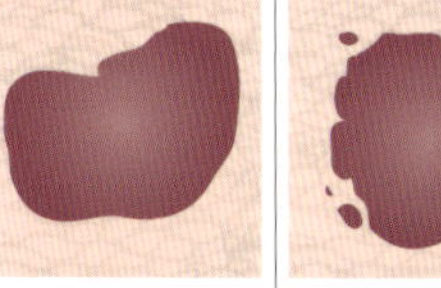	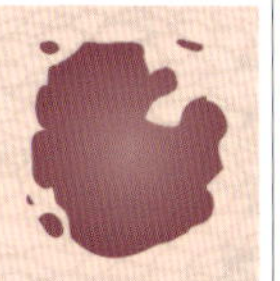	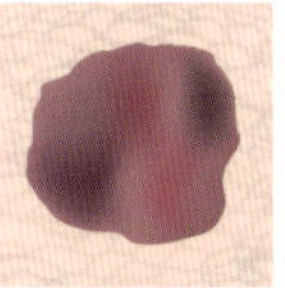	
One side of lesion does not resemble the other.	Edges irregular, ragged, notched, or blurred.	Color not uniform throughout lesion.	>6 mm or increase in size.

NCLEX Breast Self-Examination

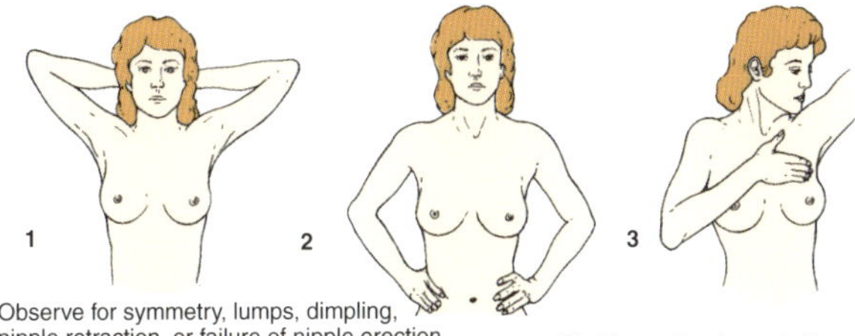

Observe for symmetry, lumps, dimpling, nipple retraction, or failure of nipple erection

Feel for nodes, irregularity, and tenderness both in breasts and in axillary areas

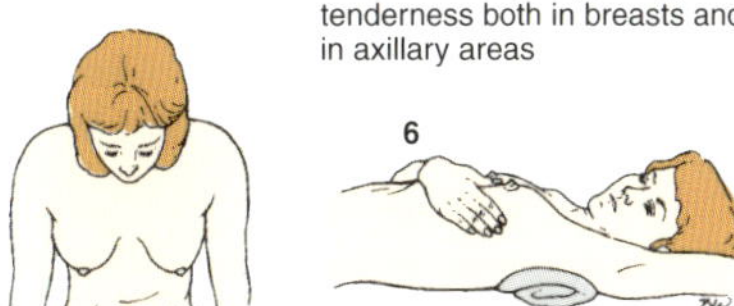

4

Gently squeeze nipple and observe for secretion, and nipple erection after each nipple is gently stimulated

While leaning forward, observe breasts as they are reflected in mirror to detect irregularity, retracted areas, nipple retraction especially on one side only

Testicular Self-Examination (TSE)

- Testicular Cancer Research Center (TCRC) recommends monthly TSE.
- Self-examination for testicular cancer is best performed after a warm bath or shower (heat relaxes the scrotum and makes it easier to spot anything abnormal).
- Stand in front of a mirror and check for any swelling on the scrotal skin.
- Examine each testicle with both hands. Place the index and middle fingers under the testicle with the thumbs placed on top.
- Roll the testicle gently between the thumbs and fingers. You should not feel pain during the examination.
- One testicle is normally slightly larger than the other.
- Find the epididymis, the soft, tubelike structure behind the testicle that collects and carries sperm. If you are familiar with this structure, you will not mistake it for a suspicious lump.
- Cancerous lumps usually are found on the sides of the testicle, but can also show up on the front.
- Lumps on the epididymis are not cancerous.

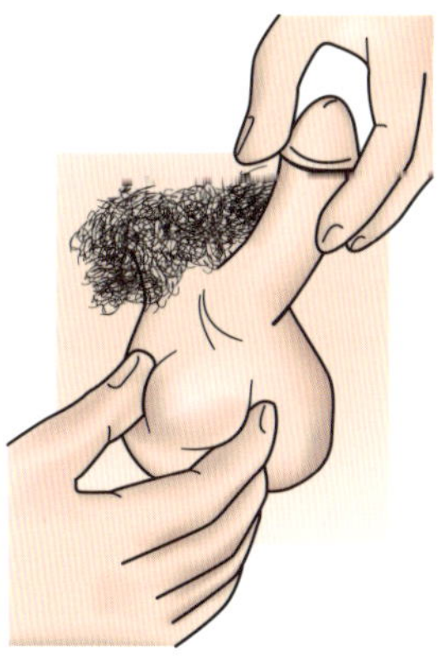

Common Types of Cancers

Breast Cancer 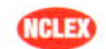

Clinical Findings: Presence of palpable breast lump, inflammation of breast, dimpling, orange-peel appearance, distended vessels, and/or nipple changes or ulcerations.

Colorectal Cancer

Clinical Findings: Changes in bowel patterns such as constipation or diarrhea, bloody stools (may be bright red or tarry in appearance), abdominal cramping, nausea and vomiting, anorexia, feeling of fullness, and palpable abdominal masses.

Hodgkin's Disease (Lymphoma)

Clinical Findings: Painless swelling of lymph nodes of neck, axillae, and inguinal areas; also fatigue, fever and chills, night sweats, unexplained weight loss, anorexia, and pruritus.

Leukemia

Clinical Findings: Fever, chills, persistent fatigue or weakness, frequent infections, anorexia, unexplained weight loss, swollen lymph nodes, enlarged liver or spleen, petechiae rash, night sweats, bone tenderness, abnormal bruising, and increased bleeding time.

Lung Cancer

Clinical Findings: Early-stage lung cancer is usually asymptomatic and discovered from abnormal findings on routine chest x-ray; advanced-stage lung cancer often manifests with persistent cough, chest pain, dyspnea, fatigue, weight loss, hemoptysis, and hoarseness.

Lymphoma

Hodgkin's disease and Non-Hodgkin's Lymphoma, this page.

Non-Hodgkin's Lymphoma (NHL)

Clinical Findings: Fatigue, unexplained weight loss, pruritus, fever, and night sweats.

Ovarian Cancer

Clinical Findings: Abdominal distention and palpable masses, unexplained weight loss, pelvic pain and discomfort, urinary urgency, and constipation.

Prostate Cancer

Clinical Findings: Possible urinary frequency, nocturia, dysuria, and hematuria. In advanced stages, Pts may complain of back pain and weight loss. Digital rectal examination reveals prostatic lesions, and lab tests show prostate-specific antigen (PSA) level > 10 ng/mL (normal is < 4 ng/mL).

Clinical Findings: Skin change (classic indication), especially new lesion with nonuniform shape and color or sore that will not heal.

Skin Cancer (Melanoma)

Clinical Findings: Change in color (usually dark blue to black), shape, or size of an existing mole or nevus.

Testicular Cancer

Clinical Findings: Earliest sign: small, hard, painless lump on testicle; other symptoms: low back pain, feeling of heaviness in scrotum, gynecomastia, and breast tenderness. Depending on stage of cancer, lymph nodes in surrounding areas may be enlarged.

Uterine Cancer

Clinical Findings: Most common symptom is abnormal, painless vaginal bleeding. Late symptoms include pain, fever, and bowel or bladder dysfunction. Palpation may reveal enlarged uterus and uterine masses. A mucosanguineous, odorous discharge may indicate vaginal metastasis.

Chronic Obstructive Pulmonary Disease (COPD)

Definition: This group of diseases causes airflow blockage and breathing-related problems. COPD includes asthma, chronic bronchitis, and emphysema. COPD is a slowly progressive disease of airways that is characterized by gradual loss of lung function.

Clinical Findings: Cough productive of sputum, shortness of breath, wheezing, and chest tightness.

Three Types of COPD

Asthma: See Asthma section (pp. 206–207).

Chronic Bronchitis: Characterized by productive cough lasting >3 months during 2 consecutive yr and airflow obstruction caused by excessive tracheobronchial mucous production.

Emphysema: Characterized by abnormal, permanent enlargement of the distal air spaces past the terminal bronchioles, loss of elasticity, distal air space distention, and alveolar septal destruction.

Nursing Focus

- Position Pt to maximize ease of breathing (HOB 30°–45°).
- Teach "pursed-lipped" breathing to decrease air trapping.
- Stage activities to conserve energy and decrease oxygen demand.
- Encourage frequent, small feedings of high-calorie foods/liquids to maximize calorie intake.
- During an exacerbation, assess and maintain ABCs, notify RT/MD, and implement collaborative care, such as meds and IV fluid, as ordered.
- Monitor vital signs, and document response to prescribed therapies.

Reinforce Patient Teaching

- Provide Pt and family with literature on specific type of COPD.
- Explain actions, dosages, side effects, and adverse reactions of meds.
- Provide instructions on proper use of metered-dose inhalers.
- Instruct Pt to seek immediate medical attention if symptoms are not relieved with prescribed meds.

Congestive Heart Failure (CHF)

Definition: Condition in which the heart is unable to pump sufficient blood to meet metabolic needs of the body. The results of inadequate cardiac output (CO) are poor organ perfusion and vascular congestion in pulmonary (left-sided failure) and systemic (right-sided failure) circulation.

Clinical Findings: Most common symptoms include fatigue, SOB, and edema (vascular congestion in either the pulmonary or systemic circulation) in ankles or feet, in sacral area, or throughout body. Ascites may cause Pt to feel bloated and may compromise respiratory effort. Onset of symptoms may be rapid or gradual, depending on underlying cause.

NCLEX ***Left-sided heart failure:*** Orthopnea, pulmonary edema, crackles or wheezes, dysrhythmias, tachycardia, tachypnea, dyspnea, anxiety, cyanosis, HTN (early CHF), low BP (late CHF), and decreased CO. NCLEX ***Right-sided heart failure:*** Dependent edema, jugular vein distention, bounding pulses, oliguria, dysrhythmias, enlargement of the liver and/or spleen, increased central venous pressure, and altered liver function tests.

Nursing Focus

- Encourage rest and help alleviate dyspnea by administering supplemental oxygen as ordered and elevating HOB 30°–45°.
- In end-stage CHF, the slightest activity can cause fatigue and SOB; therefore, assist Pt with ADLs and eating as needed. Stage activities to conserve energy and decrease oxygen demand.
- Restrict fluid intake (typically <2 L/d) and sodium intake as ordered (typically 1500–2300 mg/d depending on severity of heart failure).
- Assess vital signs before and after any level of increased activity.
- Monitor for signs and symptoms of fluid overload, impaired gas exchange, activity intolerance, daily intake and output, and weight gain to help in early detection of exacerbation.

Reinforce Patient Teaching

- Provide Pt with literature on CHF.
- Teach Pt and family to monitor for increased SOB or edema.
- Teach Pt to limit fluids to 2 L/d, and restrict sodium as ordered.
- Teach Pt to weigh self at same time every day using same scale and report any weight gain >4 lb in 2 days.

comfort that is not relieved with rest.

- Review fluid and dietary restrictions, and stress importance of reducing sodium intake.
- Explain dosages, route, actions, and adverse reactions of meds.

Coronary Artery Disease (CAD)

Definition: Narrowing and hardening of arterial lumen result in decreased coronary blood flow and decreased delivery of oxygen and nutrients to the myocardium.

Clinical Findings: Most common symptom is angina; some individuals are asymptomatic.

Nursing Focus

- Monitor vital signs and document response to prescribed therapies.
- Monitor and maintain cardiopulmonary function, and enhance myocardial perfusion by implementing prescribed therapies.
- Document nursing and medical interventions and their outcomes.

Reinforce Patient Teaching

- Provide Pt and family with literature about CAD.
- Explain lifestyle modifications necessary to control CAD.
- Review dietary restrictions and stress importance of reading food labels to avoid foods high in sodium, saturated fats, trans fats, and cholesterol.
- Explain actions, dosages, side effects, and adverse reactions of meds.
- Provide information about resumption of sexual activity acceptable for Pt's medical condition.
- If surgery is planned, provide preoperative teaching to prepare Pt and family for procedure, ICU, postoperative care, and cardiac rehabilitation.

Crohn's Disease

Definition: A type of inflammatory bowel disease (IBD), Crohn's disease usually occurs in the ileum, but it can affect any part of the digestive tract from mouth to anus. Diagnosis may be difficult, because Crohn's disease often resembles other disorders including irritable bowel syndrome (IBS) and ulcerative colitis.

Clinical Findings: Most common symptoms include abdominal pain, often in lower right quadrant, and diarrhea; rectal bleeding, weight loss, and fever are also possible; anemia is possible if bleeding persistent.

Nursing Focus

- Monitor intake and output, and maintain fluid and electrolyte balance.
- Assess for skin breakdown, and provide routine skin care.
- Unless contraindicated, fluid intake should be 3000 mL/d.
- Use calorie counts to ensure adequate nutrition.
- Monitor lab results.

Reinforce Patient Teaching

- Provide Pt and family with literature on Crohn's disease.
- Instruct Pt that fluid intake should be at least 3 L/d, and meals should be small and frequent to maintain adequate nutrition.
- Teach Pt to minimize frequency and severity of future exacerbations with adequate rest and relaxation, stress reduction or avoidance, and adequate nutrition.
- Explain dosages, route, actions, and adverse reactions of meds.

NCLEX Diabetes Mellitus (DM)

Definition: This chronic metabolic disorder is marked by hyperglycemia. DM results either from primary failure of pancreatic beta cells to produce insulin (type 1 DM) or from development of insulin resistance in body cells, with initial increased insulin secretion to maintain metabolism followed by eventual inability of pancreas to secrete enough insulin to sustain normal metabolism (type 2 DM).

Clinical Findings:

Type 1 Diabetes (previously called insulin-dependent diabetes mellitus [IDDM]): Weight loss, muscle wasting, loss of subcutaneous fat, polyuria, polydipsia, polyphagia, ketoacidosis.

Type 2 Diabetes (previously called adult-onset diabetes): Polyuria, polydipsia, pruritus, peripheral neuropathy, frequent infections, and delayed healing of wounds or sores.

Gestational Diabetes (See GERI/OB/PEDS tab.)

Nursing Focus

Assess routinely for hyperglycemia and hypoglycemia and their associated signs and symptoms.

Monitor blood glucose level as ordered, and document response to prescribed therapies.

Assess body systems for complications associated with effects of diabetes.

Reinforce Patient Teaching NCLEX

- Provide Pt with literature on managing diabetes.
- Encourage necessary lifestyle changes including weight reduction if Pt is overweight, dietary modifications, and exercise.
- Explain purpose, dosage, route, and side effects of insulin and/or oral hypo-

appropriate preparation and administration.

- Educate Pt on proper foot care to minimize risk of injury.
  - Advise Pt about importance of never going barefoot, either outside or around the house, and emphasize that soft slippers or socks do not protect against injury.
  - Instruct Pt to inspect feet every day, and use a mirror or ask someone to help if he or she has difficulty performing task alone, and to notify health-care professional of any untoward findings (e.g., cuts, skin cracks, calluses, ulcers, punctures wounds, or ingrown toenails).
  - Instruct Pt to wash feet daily, thoroughly dry, and apply moisturizing lotion to entire foot (not between toes).
  - Emphasize that Pts who have been diagnosed with diabetic neuropathy should have routine nail care performed by health-care professional or diabetic foot care specialist.

Diabetes Facts

Glucagon: Hormone secreted by alpha cells of pancreas in response to low blood sugar that increases blood glucose levels by stimulating liver to convert stored glycogen into glucose.

Glycogen: Excess carbohydrates stored in liver and muscles.

Glycosuria: Glucose present in urine, a diagnostic sign of diabetes.

Insulin: Hormone secreted by beta cells of pancreas in response to high blood glucose. Insulin is required for transport of glucose across cell membrane. Inadequate insulin level or cellular resistance to insulin results in elevated blood glucose levels (hyperglycemia).

Ketones: By-product of metabolism of fat and protein. Body responds to excess ketones (ketoacidosis) by increasing respiratory rate.

Polydipsia: Excessive thirst; diuresis causes cellular dehydration and fluid and electrolyte depletion, resulting in excessive thirst.

Polyphagia: Hunger; caused by cellular starvation, secondary to decreased amount of glucose available to cells.

Polyuria: Excessive urination; as excess glucose flows or "spills over" from kidneys, it pulls water with it by osmosis, with resulting diuresis that leads to dehydration.

NCLEX Hypertension (HTN)

Definition: HTN is persistent or intermittent elevation of SBP >140 mm Hg or DBP >90 mm Hg.

Clinical Findings:

Primary (Essential): Typically asymptomatic, primary HTN is usually not recognized until secondary complications develop (e.g., atherosclerosis, TIAs, strokes, MI, left ventricular hypertrophy, CHF, and renal failure).

Secondary: Variable, but most commonly CV and neurologic symptoms (malaise, weakness, fatigue, flushing of the face, headache, dizziness, light-headedness, nose bleeds, ringing in the ears, or blurred vision) and symptoms associated with underlying cause.

Four Stages

- **Normal BP:** SBP <120 mm Hg and DBP <80 mm Hg.
- **Prehypertension:** SBP 120–139 mm Hg or DBP 80–89 mm Hg.
- **HTN Stage I:** SBP 140–159 mm Hg or DBP 90–99 mm Hg.
- **HTN Stage II:** SBP 160 mm Hg or higher or DBP 100 mm Hg or higher.

Nursing Focus

- Monitor vital signs and document response to prescribed therapies for reducing blood pressure.
- Assess for signs of end-organ dysfunction (angina, low serum potassium levels, elevated serum creatinine and BUN, proteinuria, and uremia).
- Implement collaborative care (e.g., administering antihypertensive meds).
- **Caution:** BP must be reduced gradually; excessive and rapid reduction in BP can precipitate cerebral, myocardial, and renal ischemia.

Reinforce Patient Teaching

- Provide Pt with literature on reducing high blood pressure.
- Encourage necessary lifestyle modifications including weight reduction (for overweight Pts), limiting alcohol intake to one drink per day, increased physical activity (30–45 min/d), and smoking cessation.
- Review dietary guidelines, and stress importance of reading food labels to avoid processed foods high in sodium, saturated fats, trans fats, and cholesterol.
- Provide information to help Pt reduce intake of sodium, saturated fats, and cholesterol, and keep consumption of trans fats to an absolute minimum.
- Explain importance of maintaining adequate intake of potassium, calcium, and magnesium.
- Explain actions, dosages, side effects, and adverse reactions of HTN meds.

Irritable Bowel Syndrome (IBS)

Definition: This condition is marked by abdominal pain (often relieved by passage of stool or gas), disturbances of evacuation (constipation, diarrhea, or alternating episodes of both), bloating and abdominal distention, and passage of mucus in stools.

Clinical Findings: Classic IBS symptoms include abdominal pain, flatus, constipation, and diarrhea.

Nursing Focus

- Monitor hydration, intake, and output.
- Encourage Pt to eat small meals at regular intervals.
- Encourage fluids; goal is eight glasses of water per day.
- Encourage frequent ambulation.

Reinforce Patient Teaching

- Provide Pt and family with literature on IBS.
- Encourage necessary lifestyle changes to promote stress reduction.
- Encourage regular exercise (e.g., walking 30 min/d).
- Suggest Pt get adequate sleep and avoid becoming fatigued.
- Suggest Pt eat frequent, small meals throughout the day and avoid foods and beverages identified as triggers (e.g., wheat, barley, rye, chocolate, dairy, caffeine, or alcohol).
- Explain actions, dosages, side effects, and adverse reactions of meds.

Multiple Sclerosis (MS)

Definition: This chronic and progressive disorder of brain and spinal cord (CNS) is caused by damage to myelin sheath (white matter). Destruction of myelin sheath leads to scarring (sclerosis), which decreases and eventually blocks nerve conduction.

Clinical Findings: Weakness, paresis, or paralysis of one or more limbs, myoclonus (involuntary muscle jerks), impaired or double vision, eye and facial pain, fatigue, dizziness, decreased coordination, and loss of balance.

Nursing Focus

- Goal of therapy is to control symptoms and preserve function to maximize quality of life.
- Perform or arrange for ROM exercises to be done twice a day.
- Assess skin for breakdown and perform routine skin care.

Reinforce Patient Teaching

- Provide Pt and family with literature on MS.
- Encourage healthful and active lifestyle that includes exercise to maintain good muscle tone, good nutrition, and plenty of rest and relaxation.
- Emphasize importance of avoiding stress and fatigue.
- Depending on progression of MS, arrange for occupational, physical, and speech therapy.
- Explain actions, dosages, side effects, and adverse reactions of all meds, which may include steroids and immunosuppressant therapy, antiviral agents, muscle relaxants, and/or antidepressants.

Pancreatitis

Definition: Inflammation of pancreas is caused by activation of pancreatic enzymes within pancreas that digest pancreas itself.

Clinical Findings: Classic symptom is abdominal pain that radiates toward the back and increases when supine; other symptoms include swollen and tender abdomen that may worsen after eating, nausea, vomiting, fever, and tachycardia.

Nursing Focus

- Goals of treatment are pain management, supportive care, and prevention of secondary complications.
- Assess lab results for elevated levels of serum amylase and serum lipase.
- Monitor glucose, Ca^{++}, Mg^{++}, Na^{+}, K^{+}, and bicarbonate levels.

Reinforce Patient Teaching

- Provide Pt and family with literature on pancreatitis.
- Teach Pt to avoid alcoholic beverages and decrease consumption of foods high in fat.
- Provide teaching before diagnostic procedures, which include abdominal ultrasound to look for gallstones and CT scan to look for inflammation and destruction of pancreas.
- Explain dosages, route, actions, and adverse reactions of meds.

Peripheral Vascular Disease (PVD)

Definition: Disease of peripheral blood vessels is characterized by narrowing and hardening of arteries that supply legs and feet. Decreased blood flow results in nerve and tissue damage to extremities.

Clinical Findings: Intermittent claudication (leg pain on activity that is relieved with rest), weak or absent peripheral pulses, pallor or cyanosis, numbness, cool extremities, and minimal-to-no hair growth on extremities.

Nursing Focus

- Assess and monitor distal circulation and sensory and motor function.
- Prevent pressure sores with frequent position changes and assessment.
- Encourage and assist with frequent ambulation.

Reinforce Patient Teaching

- Provide Pt and family with literature on PVD.
- Encourage light-to-moderate activity alternated with periods of rest.
- Explain options available for smoking cessation.
- Teach Pt to reduce intake of saturated fats, trans fats, and cholesterol.

open-toed/heeled shoes), keeping feet clean and dry, and minimizing risk of injury by never going barefoot. Inspect bottom of feet daily for injuries.
- Encourage leg exercises (ankle rotations) and/or a walking regimen.
- Explain dosages, route, actions, and adverse reactions of meds.

NCLEX Renal Failure: Chronic (CRF)

Definition: CRF is a gradual and progressive loss of ability of kidneys to excrete wastes, concentrate urine, and conserve electrolytes. In contrast, acute renal failure occurs suddenly.

Clinical Findings: Edema throughout the body, SOB, fatigue, flank pain, oliguria (progressing to anuria), elevated BP, and pale skin.

Nursing Focus

- Never measure BP or perform venipuncture on an arm with a dialysis shunt.
- Help minimize discomfort from frustrations with fluid restrictions by offering ice chips, frozen lemon swabs, diversional activities, and hard candies.
- Provide routine skin care; uremia causes itching and dryness of skin.
- Monitor BUN and serum creatinine levels.
- Monitor strict fluid intake and output; fluids are typically restricted to an amount equal to previous day's urine output plus 500–600 mL.
- Perform frequent turning and ROM exercises to minimize skin breakdown.

Reinforce Patient Teaching

- Provide Pt and family with literature on CRF and/or dialysis.
- Restrict sodium, water, potassium, phosphate, and protein intake as ordered.
- Encourage compliance with secondary preventive measures.
- Explain actions, dosages, side effects, and adverse reactions of meds.

Urinary Incontinence

Definition: Intermittent or complete absence of ability to control excretion of urine.

Clinical Findings: Involuntary leakage of urine.

Types of Incontinence

Stress: Leakage of small amounts of urine during physical movement (coughing, sneezing, exercising).

Urge: Involuntary passage of urine occurring soon after a strong sense of urgency to void.

Mixed: Usually, stress and urge incontinence together.

Overflow: Unexpected leakage of urine because of a full bladder.

Functional (environmental): Untimely urination because of physical disability, external obstacles, or problems in thinking or communicating that prevent a person from reaching a toilet.

Transient: Leakage that occurs temporarily because of a condition that will pass (infection, med).

Nursing Focus

- Provide routine skin care and assessment including fluid intake and output.
- Encourage Pt to practice Kegel exercises and monitor effectiveness.
- Offer reassurance and encouragement.
- Ensure a barrier-free pathway to bathroom (functional incontinence).

Reinforce Patient Teaching

- Provide Pt and family with literature on incontinence.
- Teach Kegel exercises: Contract the pelvic floor muscles (same muscles that stop flow of urine) for 10 sec, and then relax for 10 sec. Perform 3 sets of 10 contractions every day.
- Encourage Pt to quit smoking to reduce coughing and bladder irritation. Smoking also increases risk of bladder cancer.
- Explain that alcohol and caffeine can overstimulate bladder and should be avoided.
- Advise Pt to avoid foods and drinks that may irritate bladder such as spicy foods, carbonated beverages, and citrus fruits and juices.
- Explain actions, dosages, side effects, and adverse reactions of meds.
- If surgery is planned, provide preoperative teaching to prepare Pt and family for procedure and postoperative care and recovery.

Food Sources for Specific Nutrients

Calcium-Rich Foods

- Bok choy
- Broccoli
- Canned fish
- Creamed soups
- Clams
- Dairy
- Molasses
- Oysters
- Refried beans
- Spinach
- Tofu
- Turnip greens

Iron-Rich Foods

- Cereals
- Clams
- Dried beans/peas
- Dried fruit
- Leafy green vegetables
- Lean red meat
- Molasses
- Organ meats

Potassium-Rich Foods

- Apricots
- Avocados
- Bananas
- Broccoli
- Cantaloupe
- Dried fruit
- Grapefruit
- Honey dew
- Kiwi
- Lima beans
- Meats
- Dried beans and peas
- Nuts
- Oranges
- Peaches
- Plantains
- Potatoes
- Rhubarb
- Spinach
- Sunflower seeds
- Tomatoes
- Winter squash

Sodium-Rich Foods

- Salt
- Fast food
- Canned foods
- Macaroni and cheese
- Canned sauces
- Butter
- Margarine
- Buttermilk
- Baking mixes
- Barbeque sauce
- Salad dressing
- Cured meats
- Chips
- Potato salad
- Ketchup

Low-Sodium Foods

- Baked poultry
- Canned pumpkin
- Cooked turnips
- Egg yolk
- Fresh vegetables
- Fruit
- Grits
- Honey
- Jams, jellies
- Lean meats
- Low-calorie mayonnaise
- Macaroons
- Potatoes
- Puffed wheat
- Puffed rice
- Lima beans
- Sherbet
- Unsalted nuts

Continued

Vitamin D-Rich Foods		
• Canned salmon • Canned sardines • Canned tuna	• Fish • Fish liver oils • Cereals	• Fortified milk • Nonfat dry milk

Vitamin K-Rich Foods		
• Asparagus • Beans • Broccoli • Brussels sprouts • Mustard greens	• Cauliflower • Collards • Green tea • Kale • Milk	• Cabbage • Spinach • Swiss chard • Turnips • Yogurt

Foods That Contain Tyramine		
• Aged, processed cheeses • Avocado • Bananas • Bean curd • Beer and ale • Caffeinated beverages • Caviar • Chocolate	• Distilled spirits • Sausage • Liver • Tenderized meat • Miso soup • Overripe fruit • Peanuts • Raisins • Raspberries • Red wine	• Sauerkraut • Sherry • Shrimp paste • Smoked or pickled fish • Soy sauce • Vermouth • Yeasts • Yogurts

Foods That Acidify Urine		
• Cheese • Corn • Cranberries • Eggs • Fish	• Grains • Lentils • Meats • Nuts (walnuts, Brazil nuts, filberts)	• Pasta • Plums • Poultry • Prunes • Rice

Foods That Alkalize Urine		
• All fruits except cranberries, prunes, plums	• All vegetables except corn • Milk	• Almonds • Chestnuts

Foods to Avoid With Certain Drugs/Herbs

Drug/Herb	Avoid or Moderate
Angiotensin-converting enzyme (ACE) inhibitors	Potassium-containing salt substitute
Ampicillin	Carbonated beverages, acidic juices
Aspirin	Feverfew, ginkgo, green tea
Barbiturates	Valerian
Calcium channel blockers	Grapefruit juice
Cloxacillin	Carbonated beverages, acidic juices
Cyclosporine	Grapefruit juice, potassium-containing salt substitute
Digoxin	High-fiber foods and meals
Enteric-coated pills	Excess milk, hot beverages, alcohol
Fluoroquinolones	Foods high in calcium, iron, or zinc (dairy and red meat)
Hemorrhoid medications	Saw palmetto
Indomethacin	Potassium-containing salt substitute
Isoniazid	High-carbohydrate foods
Levodopa	Excess protein
Lithium	Significant increase or decrease in sodium intake
Methyldopa	Excess protein
Monoamine oxidase inhibitors (MAOIs)	Foods that contain tyramine
NSAIDs	Asian ginseng, ginkgo
Penicillin G	Carbonated beverages, acidic juices
Phenytoin	Excess protein
Potassium-sparing diuretics	Potassium-containing salt substitute
"Statin" drugs	Grapefruit and grapefruit juice
Tetracycline	Iron-rich food or supplements, calcium
Theophylline	Excess protein
Warfarin (Coumadin)	Vitamin K-rich foods and supplements, Asian ginseng, feverfew, garlic, ginger, ginkgo, St. John's wort, green tea
Zidovudine	Excess fat

Herb–Prescription Drug Interactions

Herb	Known Drug Interaction
Aloe	Increases risks associated with cardiac glycosides.
Anise	May interfere with anticoagulants, MAOIs, and hormone therapy.
Brewer's yeast	MAOIs can cause an increase in BP.
Echinacea	May interfere with immunosuppressant agents.
Eucalyptus	Induces liver enzymes, which may increase metabolism of other drugs.
Feverfew Garlic Ginger Ginkgo	May inhibit platelet activity (avoid use with warfarin or other anticoagulants). May potentiate effects of MAOIs (ginkgo).
Ginseng	May potentiate effects of caffeine. May interfere with phenelzine. May inhibit platelet activity. (Avoid use with warfarin or other anticoagulants.)
Goldenseal	May interfere with antacids, sucralfate, H_2 antagonists, antihypertensive agents, and anticoagulants.
Hawthorne	May inhibit metabolism of ACE inhibitors and potentiate effect of cardiac glycosides.
Kava kava	May potentiate or add to effects of CNS depressants, antiplatelets, and MAOIs.
Ma-huang	Potentiates sympathomimetic effects of antihypertensives, antidepressants, and MAOIs.
Oak bark	Inhibits absorption of alkaloids and other alkaline drugs.
Peppermint	May interfere with gastric acid-blocking drugs.
Psyllium	Interferes with absorption of other drugs.
St. John's wort	May increase risk of adverse reactions to antidepressants. May significantly reduce blood concentrations of indinavir.
Saw palmetto	May interfere with oral contraceptives and hormone therapy.
Valerian	May potentiate sedative effects.

Suggested Dietary Changes Related to Diseases

Disease Process	Suggested Dietary Modification
Celiac sprue	Avoid gluten-containing foods.
Cholelithiasis	Avoid fatty foods.
Cirrhosis	Limit sodium; limit protein intake; avoid alcohol.
Congestive heart failure	Limit sodium.
Coronary artery disease	Follow American Heart Association diets.
Diabetes mellitus	Follow American Diabetic Association diet; limit calories; exercise.
Diverticulitis	Follow low-residue (low-fiber) diet.
Diverticulosis	Follow high-residue (high-fiber) diet.
Dysphagia	Use special consistency diets as indicated by testing/tolerance.
Esophagitis	Avoid alcohol, nonsteroidal drugs, tobacco; consume thick liquids.
Gastroesophageal reflux	Avoid caffeine, chocolates, mints, or late meals.
Gout	Limit alcohol, purine, and citric acid intake.
Hyperhomocysteinemia	Increase consumption of folates and vitamin B_{12}.
Hyperlipidemias	Follow National Cholesterol Education Program diet with limited fat and cholesterol, and increased fiber.
Iron-deficiency anemia	Take iron supplements with vitamin C.
Irritable bowel syndrome	Increase fiber content of meals; limit dairy products.
Kidney stone formers	Ensure liberal fluid intake.
Nephrotic syndrome	Limit sodium intake.
Obesity	Restrict calories, increase exercise.
Osteoporosis	Supplement calcium and vitamin D; limit alcohol and tobacco.
Pernicious anemia	Supplement cyanocobalamin (vitamin B_{12}).
Renal failure	Limit sodium, potassium, protein, and fluids.
Women and men, >25 yr	Supplement calcium: 1000 mg/d (1200 mg/d if >50 yr old).

Common Formulas and Equivalents

Body Surface Area (BSA) Formula

Using cm and kg	Using in and lb
$\sqrt{[(\text{height} \times \text{weight}) \div 3600]}$	$\sqrt{[(\text{height} \times \text{weight}) \div 3131]}$

Common Equivalents

Volume		Weight	
1 cc	1 mL	1 mg	1000 mcg
1 tsp	5 mL	1 g	1000 mg
1 tbsp	15 mL	1 kg	1000 g
1 oz	30 mL	1 gr	60 mg
1 c	240 mL	1/150 gr	0.4 mg
1 pt	473 mL	1 kg	2.2 lb
1 qt	946 mL	1 L	1 kg
1 L	960 oz	1 oz	28 g

Common Standard-to-Metric Formulas

	Standard	Metric
Weight	lb = kg × 2.2	kg = lb × 0.45 or (lb ÷ 2) – 10%
Temp	°F = (°C × 1.8) + 32	°C = (°F × 32) ÷ 1.8
Volume	oz to mL = oz × 30	mL to oz = mL ÷ 30
Length	in. = cm × 0.394	cm = in. × 2.54

Waist-to-Hip Ratio

Desired Waist-to-Hip Ratio: Women Up to 0.8; Men Up to 0.95

1. Measure circumference of waist at narrowest point with stomach relaxed.
2. Measure circumference of hips at fullest point where buttocks protrude most.
3. Divide circumference of waist by circumference of hips.

Conversions: Standard-to-Metric

Weight		Temp		Height	
lb	kg	°F	°C	in.	cm
325	148	212	100 boil	50 (4′2″)	127
300	136	107	41.7	51 (4′3″)	130
275	125	106.7	41	52 (4′4″)	132
250	114	105	40.6	53 (4′5″)	135
225	102	104	40	54 (4′6″)	137
210	96	103	39.4	55 (4′7″)	140
200	91	102	38.9	56 (4′8″)	142
190	86	101	38.3	57 (4′9″)	145
180	82	100.4	38	58 (4′10″)	147
170	77	100	37.7	59 (4′11″)	150
160	73	99.6	37.5	60 (5′)	152
150	68	98.6	37.0	61 (5′1″)	155
140	64	98	36.7	62 (5′2″)	157
130	59	97.7	36.5	63 (5′3″)	160
120	55	96.8	36	64 (5′4″)	163
110	50	95.9	35.5	65 (5′5″)	165
100	46	95	35	66 (5′6″)	168
90	41	94.1	34.5	67 (5′7″)	170
80	36	93.2	34	68 (5′8″)	173
70	32	91.4	33	69 (5′9″)	175
60	27	89.6	32	70 (5′10″)	178
50	23	87.8	31	71 (5′11″)	180
40	18	86	30	72 (6′)	183
30	14	82.4	28	73 (6′1″)	185
25	11	78.8	26	74 (6′2″)	188
20	9	75.2	24	75 (6′3″)	191
15	7	71.6	22	76 (6′4″)	193
10	4.5	68	20	77 (6′5″)	196
5	2.3	32	0 freeze	78 (6′6″)	199

Cultural Diversity in Health Care

Selected Reference: Purnell, L., & Paulanka, B. (2005). *Guide to Culturally Competent Health Care.* Philadelphia, PA: F.A. Davis.

NCLEX American Indian

Communication: Greetings should be formal. Long periods of silence are normal. Talking loud is rude. Physical contact from strangers is unacceptable; however, shaking hands is okay. Personal space is generally greater by conventional U.S. standards.

Health-Care Practices: Extensive questioning during an assessment may foster mistrust. Most individuals are stoic by conventional U.S. standards and believe that pain should be endured. Common practices include use of medicinal herbs, traditional healers, and maintenance of balance between tribal members and the universe.

Taboos and Disrespect: Direct eye contact and pointing are avoided. Physical contact with the dead is prohibited in some tribes.

Arab Heritage

Communication: Speech may be loud and expressive; it may involve gesturing, with an emphasis on nonverbal communication; avoid misinterpreting as anger or confrontation. Title is important; ask how Pt or family prefers to be addressed. Shaking hands (right hand only) is accepted, but men should not initiate a handshake with a woman.

Health-Care Practices: Same-sex health-care provider is strongly preferred. Pts are reluctant to share sensitive medical information with strangers. Most individuals are stoic; take cues from family members regarding Pt discomfort.

Taboos and Disrespect: The left hand is used for toileting and is considered dirty. Direct eye contact between members of the opposite sex may be considered disrespectful.

NCLEX Asian Heritage

Note: *C, J, K,* and *V* refer to *Chinese, Japanese, Korean,* and *Vietnamese.*

Communication: Greetings should be formal (C, J, K, V). Direct eye contact (C, J, K) or invasion of personal space (C, J) may cause uneasiness. Touch only when necessary (C, J, V). Shaking hands is accepted (J, K), but men should not initiate a handshake with women (V).

women (C, K, V). Pts may seek traditional, alternative treatment first before accepting Western medicine (C, J, K, V) and may be reluctant to accept pain medication (J, K).

Taboos and Disrespect: These include open discussion about serious illness and death (J), addiction (J), mental illness, (J), NCLEX direct eye contact (C, J, V), pointing (V), and NCLEX touching the head (V).

Bosnian Heritage

Communication: Older and traditional Pts expect formal greetings. Women maintain eye contact with other women but not with men. Physical contact between sexes is not exhibited in public. Shaking hands (right hand only) is accepted, but men should not initiate handshake with women. Asking too many questions may cause apprehension.

Health-Care Practices: High value is placed on cleanliness. Same-sex health-care provider is strongly preferred. Most individuals are stoic by Western standards; take cues from family regarding Pt discomfort.

Taboos and Disrespect: The left hand is used for toileting and is considered dirty.

Cuban Heritage

Communication: Speech tends to be loud and fast by conventional U.S. standards. Direct eye contact is acceptable during conversation. Greetings should be formal. Handshakes and casual contact are accepted, but physical contact during an assessment may need to be explained.

Health-Care Practices: Language is the biggest barrier to health care, and many Pts may seek traditional, alternative treatment first; otherwise, conventional modern medicine is openly accepted. Pain is expressed openly as verbal complaints, moaning, and crying.

Taboos and Disrespect: None noted.

Filipino Heritage

Communication: Adults should be greeted formally. Prolonged eye contact is avoided with a figure of authority or elders. Meanings are embedded in nonverbal communication. Male health-care workers should avoid prolonged eye contact with younger female Pts. Close, personal space should be respected.

Health-Care Practices: High value is placed on personal cleanliness. Pts may seek traditional, alternative treatment first. They are stoic by Western standards and may refuse pain medication.

Taboos and Disrespect: None noted.

Haitian Heritage

Communication: Greetings should be formal, and shaking hands is accepted. Haitians are very expressive with their emotions, and their speech is loud and animated. Do not misinterpret loud speech as anger. Eye contact with authority figures is avoided, but otherwise is acceptable. Casual touching is a common gesture and is not considered inappropriate.

Health-Care Practices: Haitians often use traditional and conventional modern practitioners simultaneously. Privacy is highly regarded; therefore, family should not be used for interpretation. Pain manifests outwardly with moaning and facial expressions. Many Pts have a very low pain threshold.

Taboos and Disrespect: None noted.

NCLEX Mexican Heritage

Communication: Emphasis is placed on verbal communication. Greetings should be formal. Older generations may regard direct eye contact as disrespectful, but many younger persons do not. Shaking hands is accepted, but physical contact during assessment may need to be explained.

Health-Care Practices: Assumption of the sick role is highly tolerated by family. You may need to explain pain medication.

Taboos and Disrespect: Direct eye contact with older persons is avoided.

Puerto Rican Heritage

Communication: Speech is fast by U.S. standards. Greetings should be formal. Older generations may regard direct eye contact as disrespectful, but many younger persons encourage it. Shaking hands is encouraged. Older women may require more personal space when interacting with men.

Health-Care Practices: Women may need to consult husband before signing consent. Pts may request same-sex health-care provider. Many combine traditional, folk, and conventional modern medicine. Many Pts tend to be loud and outspoken when expressing pain. Pain medication is openly accepted. Older generations may not understand the concept of a pain scale.

Taboos and Disrespect: Addressing Pt or family with terms such as "honey" may be considered disrespectful. Refusing food from family members may be regarded as personal rejection.

ussian Heritage

Communication: Greetings should be formal. Direct eye contact and touching are acceptable, independent of age and sex. Until trust is established, Pts may be standoffish toward EMS.

Health-Care Practices: Cupping is a form of suction cup–like therapy used to treat many respiratory illnesses. It produces bruising on the back that may be misinterpreted as a sign of abuse. Pts are stoic by Western standards and are not likely to ask for or accept pain medication.

Taboos and Disrespect: None noted.

English-to-Spanish Translation

English phrase • [pro-nun-ci-a-tion] • Spanish phrase

Introductions: Greetings

- **Hello** [**oh**-lah] Hola
- **Good morning** [**bweh**-nohs **dee**-ahs] Buenos días
- **Good afternoon** [**bweh**-nahs **tahr**-dehs] Buenas tardes
- **Good evening** [**bweh**-nahs **noh**-chehs] Buenas noches
- **My name is** [meh **yah**-moh] Me llamo
- **I am a nurse** [soy lah oon en-fehr-**meh**-ra] Soy la enfermera
- **What is your name?** [**koh**-moh seh **yah**-mah oo-**sted**?] ¿Cómo se llama usted?
- **How are you?** [**koh**-moh eh-**stah** oo-**stehd**?] ¿Cómo está usted?
- **Very well** [mwee **b'yehn**] Muy bien
- **Thank you** [**grah**-s'yahs] Gracias
- **Yes, No** [**see**, **noh**] Sí, No
- **Please** [pohr fah-**vohr**] Por favor
- **You're welcome** [deh **nah**-dah] De nada

Assessment: Areas of the Body

- **Head** [kah-**beh**-sah] Cabeza
- **Eye** [**oh**-hoh] Ojo
- **Ear** [oh-**ee**-doh] Oído
- **Nose** [nah-**reez**] Nariz
- **Throat** [gahr-**gahn**-tah] Garganta
- **Neck** [**kweh**-yoh] Cuello
- **Chest, Heart** [**peh**-choh, kah-rah-**sohn**] Pecho, corazón
- **Back** [eh-**spahl**-dah] Espalda
- **Abdomen** [ahb-**doh**-mehn] Abdomen

- **Stomach** [eh-**stoh**-mah-goh] Estómago
- **Rectum** [**rehk**-toh] Recto
- **Penis** [**peh**-neh] Pene
- **Vagina** [vah-**hee**-nah] Vagina
- **Arm** [**brah**-soh] Brazo
- **Hand** [**mah**-noh] Mano
- **Leg** [**p'yehr**-nah] Pierna
- **Foot** [**p'yeh**] Pie

Assessment: History

Do you have... [**T'yeh**-neh oo-**stehd**...] ¿Tiene usted...

- Difficulty breathing? [di-fi-kul-**thad pah**-reh reh-spee-**rahr**] ¿Dificultad para respirar?
- Chest pain? [doh-**lorh** hen el **peh**-chow] ¿Dolor en el pecho?
- Abdominal pain? [doh-**lorh** ab-do-mee-**nahl**] ¿Dolor abdominal?
- Diabetes? [dee-ah-**beh**-tehs] ¿Diabetes?

Are you... [¿ehs-**tah**...] ¿Está...

- Dizzy? [¿mar-eh-**a**-dho(dha)?] ¿Mareado(a)?
- Nauseated? [¿kohn **now**-say-as?] ¿Con nauseas?
- Pregnant? [¿ehm-bah-rah-**sah**-dah?] ¿Embarazada?

Are you allergic to any medications? [¿ehs ah-**lehr**-hee-koh ah ahl-**goo**-nah meh-dee-**see**-nah?] ¿Es alergico a alguna medicina?

Assessment: Pain

Do you have pain? [**T'yeh**-neh oo-**stehd** doh-**lorh**?] ¿Tiene usted dolor? [(0) cero, (1) uno, (2) dos, (3) tres, (4) cuatro, (5) cinco, (6) seis, (7) siete, (8) ocho, (9) nueve, (10) diez]

Where does it hurt? [dohn-deh leh **dweh**-leh?] ¿Donde le duele?

Is the pain... [es oon doh-**lor**...] ¿Es un dolor...

- Dull? [**Leh**-veh] ¿Leve?
- Aching? [kans-**tan**-teh] ¿Constante?
- Crushing? [ah-plahs-**than**-teh?] ¿Aplastante?
- Sharp? [ah-**goo**-doh?] ¿Agudo?
- Stabbing? [ah-**poo**-neo-lawn-teh] ¿Apuñalante?
- Burning? [Ahr-**d'yen**-teh?] ¿Ardiente?

Does it hurt when I press here? [Leh dweh-**leh** kwahn-doh leh ah-pree-**eh**-toh ah-**kee**?] ¿Le duele cuando le aprieto aqui?

Does it hurt to breathe deeply? [S'yen-teh oo-**sted** doh-lor kwahn-doh reh-**spee**-rah pro-foon-dah-**men**-teh?] ¿Siente usted dolor cuando respira profundamente?

Does it move to another area? [Leh doh-**lor** zeh moo-eh-veh a **oh**-thra ah-ri-ah] ¿El dolor se mueve a otra area?

Is the pain better now? [**S'yen**-teh al-**goo**-nah me-horr-**ee**-ah] ¿Siente alguna

Symbols and Abbreviations

ā before
α alpha
β beta
@ at
# pound, quantity
" inch
Ⓡ right
Ⓛ left
Ⓑ bilateral
↑ increase
↓ decrease
ψ psychiatric
Ø none, no
Δ change
/ per or divided by
< less than
> greater than
° degrees
Rx treatment, prescription
μ micro
AAA abdominal aortic aneurysm
ABC automated blood count (airway, breathing, circulation)
ABD abdominal (dressing)
ABG arterial blood gas
AC before meals (a.m.), antecubital
ACE angiotensin-converting enzyme
ACLS advanced cardiac life support
ACS acute coronary syndrome
ACTH adrenocorticotropin hormone
AD right ear, Alzheimer's disease
ADA American Diabetes Association
ADH antidiuretic hormone
ADHD attention deficit/hyperactivity disorder
ADLs activities of daily living
ADR adverse drug reaction
AED automated external defibrillator
AHA American Heart Association
AIDS acquired immunodeficiency syndrome
AKA above knee amputation
ALOC altered level of consciousness
ALS advanced life support, amyotrophic lateral sclerosis
AMI acute myocardial infarction
AMPLE see SAMPLE
AMS altered mental status, acute mountain sickness
AP anterior to posterior
APAP abbreviation for acetaminophen, Tylenol
APGAR appearance, pulse, grimace, activity, respiration
aPTT activated partial thromboplastin time
AS left ear
ASA abbreviation for aspirin
AU both ears
AV atrioventricular
AVB atrioventricular block
AVM arteriovenous malformation
AVPU alert, verbal, painful, unresponsive
BBB bundle branch block
BCC, BCCa basal cell carcinoma
BE barium enema, base excess
bid twice a day
BKA below knee amputation
BM bowel movement
BMI body mass index
BP blood pressure
BPH benign prostatic hyperplasia
BPM beats per minute
BS blood sugar, bowel sounds
BSA body *or* burn surface area
BUN blood urea nitrogen
BVM bag-valve mask
c̄ with
°C degrees Celsius, centigrade
C & S or CS culture and sensitivity
Ca^{++} calcium
CA cancer
CAD coronary artery disease

CBC complete blood count
CBG chemical blood glucose
CDC Centers for Disease Control and Prevention
CF cystic fibrosis
CHB complete heart block
CHF congestive heart failure
CI cardiac index
Cl^- chloride
CNS central nervous system
CO carbon monoxide, cardiac output
CO_2 carbon dioxide
COPD chronic obstructive pulmonary disease
CP chest pain, cerebral palsy
CPAP continuous positive airway pressure
CPR cardiopulmonary resuscitation
CSF cerebrospinal fluid
CSM circulation sensory and motor
CT computed tomography
CV cardiovascular
CVA cerebrovascular accident
CVC central venous catheter
CVP central venous pressure
Cx circumflex coronary artery
D5W 5% dextrose in water
DBP diastolic blood pressure
DC discontinue, direct current
DIC disseminated intravascular coagulopathy
DKA diabetic ketoacidosis
dL deciliter
DM diabetes mellitus
DOPE dislodgment, obstruction, pneumothorax, equipment
DT delirium tremens
DTS distance, time, shielding
DVT deep vein thrombosis
DZ, Dz disease
ECG or EKG electrocardiogram
ED erectile dysfunction, emergency department (ER)
EFM electronic fetal monitoring
EMS emergency medical services
EPS extrapyramidal symptoms
ESR erythrocyte sedimentation rate
ET endotracheal
ETOH abbreviation for alcohol
ETT endotracheal tube
°F degrees Fahrenheit
F and E fluid and electrolytes
Fe iron
FFP fresh frozen plasma
FHR fetal heart rate
Fr, fr French
GCS Glasgow Coma Scale
GI gastrointestinal
gtt drop
GU genitourinary
H & H hemoglobin and hematocrit
h, hr hour
H^+ hydrogen ion
HA headache
HACE high-altitude cerebral edema
HAPE high-altitude pulmonary edema
HAZMAT hazardous material
HB heart block
HCl hydrogen chloride
HCO_3 carbonic acid
Hct hematocrit
HCTZ hydrochlorothiazide
HELLP hemolysis, elevated liver enzymes, low platelets
Hgb homoglobin
HHNS hyperglycemic, hyperosmolar, nonketotic syndrome
HIV human immunodeficiency virus
HOB head of bed
HRT hormone replacement therapy
HS hour of sleep (nighttime)
HTN hypertension
HVS hyperventilation syndrome
IBC iron binding capacity
IBD irritable bowel disease
IBS irritable bowel syndrome
IBW ideal body weight
IC incident commander
ICP intracranial pressure
ICS intercostal space

IDDM insulin-dependent diabetes mellitus
IHSS idiopathic hypertrophic subaortic stenosis
IM intramuscular
IN intranasal
INH abbreviation for isoniazid
INR international normalized ratio
IO intraosseous
I/O intake and output
IV intravenous
IVC inferior vena cava
IVF Intravenous fluid
IVP Intravenous push
IVPB Intravenous piggyback
J joule
JVD jugular vein distention
K^+ potassium
KB knife blade (scalpel)
KCl potassium chloride
kg kilogram
LAD left anterior descending
LAT lateral
LBBB left bundle branch block
LLQ left lower quadrant
LMA laryngeal mask airway
LNMP last normal menstrual period
LOC level of consciousness
LPM liters per minute
LR lactated Ringer's (solution)
LTC left to count
LUQ left upper quadrant
mA milliampere
MAOI monoamine oxidase inhibitor
MAP mean arterial pressure
MAR medication administration record
MAST military antishock trousers
MCA motorcycle accident
mcg microgram
MCI mass casualty incident
MCL modified chest lead
mEq milliequivalent
mg milligram
$MgSO_4$ magnesium sulfate
MH malignant hyperthermia
MI myocardial infarction
min minute, minimum
mL milliliter
mm millimeter
mm Hg millimeter of mercury
MRI magnetic resonance imaging
MRSA methicillin-resistant *Staphylococcus aureus*
MS morphine sulfate, multiple sclerosis, musculoskeletal
MSO_4 morphine sulfate
MVA motor vehicle accident
Na^+ sodium
NAD no apparent/acute distress
$NaHCO_3$ sodium bicarbonate
NG nasogastric
NGT nasogastric tube
NI nasointestinal
NIDDM non–insulin-dependent diabetes mellitus
NPA nasopharyngeal airway
NPO nothing by mouth
NRB nonrebreather
NS normal saline
NSAID nonsteroidal anti-inflammatory drug
NSR normal sinus rhythm
NTG nitroglycerin
NTP nitroglycerin paste
n/v nausea and vomiting
O_2 oxygen
OCD obsessive compulsive disorder
OD overdose, right eye
OLMC online medical control
OPA oropharyngeal airway
OPP organophosphate
OPQRST onset, provocation, quality, radiation, severity, timing
OS left eye
OT occupational therapy
OTC over the counter
OU both eyes

oz ounce
p̄ after
PAC premature atrial complex
PAD peripheral artery disease
PaO_2 partial pressure of oxygen in arterial blood
PAP pulmonary artery pressure
PASG pneumatic antishock garment
PCI percutaneous intervention
PCW pulmonary capillary wedge pressure
PDA patent ductus arteriosus
PE pulmonary embolism, edema
PEA pulseless electrical activity
PEEP positive end-expiratory pressure
PERRL pupils equal, round and reactive to light
PET positron emission tomography
PFIB perfluoroisobutene
pH potential of hydrogen
PICC peripherally inserted central catheter
PIH pregnancy-induced hypertension
PJC premature junctional complex
PMI point of maximal impulse
PMS premenstrual syndrome
PO per os (by mouth, orally)
PPD purified protein derivative (tuberculosis skin test)
PPE personal protective equipment
PPF plasma protein fraction
PPV positive pressure ventilation
PQRST see OPQRST
PRBC packed red blood cells
PRI PR interval
prn as needed
PSA prostate-specific antigen
PSI pounds per square inch
PSVT paroxysmal supraventricular tachycardia
Pt patient
PT prothrombin time, physical therapy
PTSD posttraumatic stress disorder
PTT partial thromboplastin time
PVC premature ventricular complex
PVD peripheral vascular disease
q, Q every
qid four times per day
qod every other day
R regular (insulin)
RA rheumatoid arthritis
RBBB right bundle branch block
RCA right coronary artery
RL Ringer's lactate (solution)
RLQ right lower quadrant
ROM range of motion, rupture of membranes
RR respiratory rate
RSI rapid sequence intubation
RSV respiratory syncytial virus
RT respiratory therapy, right
RTS revised trauma score
RUQ right upper quadrant
s̄ without
SAMPLE signs and symptoms, allergies, medications, pertinent history, last oral intake, events leading up
SaO_2 oxygen saturation
SBP systolic blood pressure
SC or SQ subcutaneous
SCC squamous cell carcinoma
SI stroke index
SLP speech language pathology
SLUDGEM salivate, lacrimate, urinate, defecate, gastrointestinal distress, emesis, miosis or muscle twitching
SOB shortness of breath
SpO_2 pulse oximeter
ss, s/s signs and symptoms
STD sexually transmitted disease
SV stroke volume
SVC superior vena cava
SVR systemic venous resistance
T temperature
TB tuberculosis

TCA tricyclic antidepressant
TCP transcutaneous pacing
TF tube feeding
TIA transient ischemic attack
tid three times per day
TKO to keep open (30 mL/hr)
TPN total parenteral nutrition
TPR temperature, pulse, respirations
TVP transvenous pacing
u, U unit
UA urinalysis
UC ulcerative colitis
UO urine output
UTI urinary tract infection
VAD vascular access device
VF ventricular fibrillation
VRE vancomycin-resistant *Enterococcus*
VRSA vancomycin-resistant *Staphylococcus aureus*
VT ventricular tachycardia
WBC white blood count
WC wheel chair
WMD weapons of mass destruction
WPW Wolff-Parkinson White (syndrome)

Web Resources

Agency for Healthcare Research and Quality: http://www.ahrq.gov
American Academy of Ophthalmology: http://www.aao.org/aao/
American Cancer Society: http://www.cancer.org
American Dental Association: http://www.ada.org
American Diabetes Association: http://www.diabetes.org
American Dietetic Association: http://www.eatright.org
American Heart Association: http://www.heart.org/HEARTORG
American Holistic Nurses Association: http://www.ahna.org
American Lung Association: http://www.lung.org
American Pain Society: http://www.americanpainsociety.org/
Centers for Disease Control and Prevention: http://www.cdc.gov/
Department of Health and Human Services: http://www.hhs.gov/
Healthy People: http://www.healthypeople.gov
Infusion Nurses Society: http://www.ins1.org
National Association for Practical Nurse Education and Service: http://www.napnes.org/index.html
National Cancer Institute: http://www.cancer.gov/
National Center for Complementary and Alternative Medicine: http://nccam.nih.gov/
National Eye Institute: http://www.nei.nih.gov/
National Federation of LPNs: http://www.nflpn.org/
National Heart, Lung and Blood Institute: http://www.nhlbi.nih.gov/
National Human Genome Research Institute: http://www.genome.gov/
National Institute of Allergy and Infectious Diseases: http://www.niaid.nih.gov/
National Institute of Arthritis and Musculoskeletal and Skin Diseases: http://www.niams.nih.gov/

National Institute of Child Health and Human Development: http://www.nichd.nih.gov/

National Institute of Dental and Craniofacial Research: http://www.nidcr.nih.gov/

National Institute of Diabetes and Digestive and Kidney Diseases: http://www2.niddk.nih.gov/

National Institute of Environmental Health Sciences: http://www.niehs.nih.gov/

National Institute of General Medical Sciences: http://www.nigms.nih.gov/

National Institutes of Health: http://www.health.nih.gov

National Institute of Mental Health: http://www.nimh.nih.gov/

National Institute of Neurological Disorders and Stroke: http://www.ninds.nih.gov/

National Institute of Nursing Research: http://www.ninr.nih.gov/

National Institute on Aging: http://www.nia.nih.gov/

National Institute on Alcohol Abuse and Alcoholism: http://www.niaaa.nih.gov/

National Institute on Deafness and Other Communication Disorders: http://www.nidcd.nih.gov/

National Institute on Drug Abuse: http://www.drugabuse.gov/

National Institute on Minority Health and Health Disparities: http://www.nimhd.nih.gov/

National Library of Medicine: http://www.nlm.nih.gov/

Mental Health America: http://www.mentalhealthamerica.net/

United States Department of Agriculture: http://www.usda.gov

United States Department of Agriculture Choose My Plate: http://www.choosemyplate.gov/

Wound Ostomy and Continence Nurses Society: http://www.wocn.org

Select References

American Heart Association. (2010). 2010 American Heart Association Guidelines for CPR and ECC. *Circulation, 122*(18, Suppl. 3).

Deglin, J. H., & Vallerand, A. H. (2009). *Davis's drug guide for nurses* (11th ed.). Philadelphia, PA: FA Davis.

Dillon, P. M. (2004). *Nursing health assessment: Clinical pocket guide*. Philadelphia, PA: FA Davis.

Dubin, D. (2000). *Rapid interpretation of EKG's* (6th ed.). Tampa, FL: Cover Publishing Company.

Elkin, M. K., Perry, A. G., & Potter, P. A. (2004). *Nursing interventions and clinical skills* (3rd ed.). St. Louis, MO: Mosby Inc.

Hazinski, M. F., Samson, R., & Schexnayder, S. (Eds.). (2010). *2010 handbook of emergency cardiovascular care for healthcare providers*. Dallas, TX: American Heart Association.

(2nd ed.). Philadelphia, PA: FA Davis.

http://wonder.cdc.gov/wonder/prevguid/p0000419/p0000419.asp **(standard precautions)**

http://www.cdc.gov/ncidod/hip/isolat/isotab_1.htm **(standard precautions)**

http://www.emedicine.com/EMERG/topic25.htm **(anaphylaxis)**

http://www.emedicine.com/emerg/topic554.htm **(seizures)**

http://www.emedicine.com/emerg/topic603.htm **(transfusion Reactions)**

http://www.fpnotebook.com/ER92.htm **(oxygen delivery equipment)**

http://www.jointcommission.org/NR/rdonlyres/2329F8F5-6EC5-4E21-B932-54B2B7D53F00/0/dnu_list.pdf **(the joint commission official do not use list – 2009)**

http://www.nlm.nih.gov/medlineplus/ency/article/000009.htm **(child birth)**

http://www.nlm.nih.gov/medlineplus/ency/article/003430.htm **(serum theophylline and propranolol level)**

http://www.rcsed.ac.uk/journal/vol45_3/4530010.htm **(sepsis and SIRS)**

Johnson, J. Y., & Smith Temple, J. (2010). *Nurses' guide to clinical procedures* (6th ed.). Philadelphia, PA: Lippincott Williams & Wilkins.

Leonard, M., Bonacum, D., & Graham, S. (2013). SBAR technique for communication: A situational briefing model. Cambridge, MA: Institute for Health Care Improvement.

Lipman, B. C., & Cascio, T. (1994). *ECG: Assessment and interpretation.* Philadelphia, PA: FA Davis.

LPN expert guides: Advanced skills. (2007). Philadelphia, PA: Lippincott Williams & Wilkins.

Lutz, C., & Przytulski, K. (2004). *Nutri notes: Nutrition and diet therapy pocket guide.* Philadelphia, PA: FA Davis.

Lynn, P. (2011). *Taylor's handbook of clinical nursing skills.* Philadelphia, PA: Wolters Kluwer Health / Lippincott Williams & Wilkins.

McKinney, E. S. (2000). *Maternal-child nursing.* Philadelphia, PA: Saunders.

Perry, A. G., & Potter, P. A. (2011). *Mosby's pocket guide to nursing skills and procedures* (7th ed.). St. Louis, MO: Mosby Inc.

Purnell, L. (2009). *Guide to culturally competent health care* (2nd ed.). Philadelphia, PA: F.A. Davis.

Rosen, P., Barkin, R. M., Schaider, J. J., Hayden, S. R., & Wolfe, R. E. (Eds.). (2003). *Rosen and Barkin's 5-minute emergency medicine consult* (2nd ed.). Philadelphia, PA: Lippincott Williams & Wilkins.

Silvestri, L. A. (2010). *Saunders comprehensive review for the NCLEX-PN examination* (4th ed.). St. Louis, MO: Saunders Elsevier.

Silvestri, L. A. (2008). *Saunders comprehensive review for the NCLEX-RN examination* (4th ed.). St. Louis, MO: Saunders Elsevier.

Singer, A. J., Burstein, J. L., & Schiavone, F. M. (2001). *Emergency medicine pearls* (2nd ed.). Philadelphia, PA: FA Davis.

Sommers, M. S. (2011). *Diseases and disorders: A nursing therapeutics manual* (4th ed.). Philadelphia, PA: FA Davis.

Townsend, M. C. (2003). *Psychiatric mental health nursing: Concepts of care* (4th ed.). Philadelphia, PA: FA Davis.

Townsend, M. C. (2004). *Nursing diagnoses in psychiatric nursing: Care plans and psychotropic medications* (6th ed.). Philadelphia, PA: FA Davis.

Van Leeuwen, A. M., & Poelhuis-Leth, D. J. (2009). *Davis's comprehensive handbook of laboratory and diagnostic tests with nursing implications* (3rd ed.). Philadelphia, PA: FA Davis.

Venes, D. (Ed.). (2009). *Taber's cyclopedic medical dictionary* (21st ed.). Philadelphia, PA: FA Davis.

Illustration Checklist Report

Pages 2, 116 (top left and right) from Williams, L. S., & Hopper, P. D. (2003). *Understanding medical surgical nursing* (2nd ed.). Philadelphia, PA: FA Davis.

Pages 3, 5, 52, 74, 180 from Wilkinson, J. M., & Treas, L. M. (2010). *Fundamentals of nursing* (Vol. 1; 2nd ed.). Philadelphia, PA: FA Davis.

Pages 8, 9, 20, 22, 35, 38–41, 45 from Burton, M., & Ludwig, L. (2010). *Fundamentals of nursing care: Concepts, connections, and skills.* Philadelphia, PA: FA Davis.

Pages 12, 13 from Myers, E., & Hale, A. (2013). *RN PocketPro*. Philadelphia, PA: FA Davis.

Page 65 from Hockenberry, M. J., & Wilson, D. (2009). *Wong's essentials of pediatric nursing* (8th ed.). St. Louis, MO: Mosby.

Page 92 from Chapman, L., & Durham, R. (2009). *Maternal newborn nursing: The critical components of nursing care*. Philadelphia, PA: FA Davis.

Pages 116 (bottom right), 208, 210 from Myers, E., & Hopkins, T. (2007). *LPN notes: Nurse's clinical pocket guide* (2nd ed.). Philadelphia, PA: FA Davis.

Page 117 (top left, middle left and right) from Myers, E., & Hopkins, T. (2007). *MedSurg notes: Nurse's clinical pocket guide* (2nd ed.). Philadelphia, PA: FA Davis.

Pages 117 (bottom right), 123, 155, 205 (last strip) from Myers, E. (2009). *EMS notes: EMT & paramedic field guide*. Philadelphia, PA: FA Davis.

Page 135 from Singer, A. J., Burstein, J. L., & Schiavone, F. M. (2001). *Emergency medicine pearls* (2nd ed.). Philadelphia, PA: FA Davis.

Pages 175, 177, 199 (top left and right), 201–204, 205 (top three) from Myers, E. (2012). *LPN notes: Nurse's clinical pocket guide* (3rd ed.). Philadelphia, PA: FA Davis.

Page 197 from Jones, S. A. (2009). *ECG notes: Interpretation and management guide* (2nd ed.). Philadelphia, PA: FA Davis.

Page 209 from Venes, D. (Ed.). (2009). Taber's cyclopedic medical dictionary (21st ed.). Philadelphia, PA: FA Davis.

Index

Note: Page numbers followed by "f" and "t" indicate figures and tables, respectively.

- Vital clinical information
- Portable and pocket-sized
- Easy-to-reference tabs
- HIPAA-compliant

Deliver safe and effective health care!
Access the clinically oriented content you need to deliver safe and effective health care in hospital and home settings. *Plus,* NCLEX tips, highlighted throughout, make this the perfect pocket-sized resource for those preparing for the licensure exam.

NEW TO THIS EDITION

- **NEW! Streamlined organization**
- **NEW! "Nursing Alerts"** that highlight safety information.
- **NEW! SBAR** Communication Technique.
- **NEW!** Coverage of wound cultures • condom catheters • assessment overview • sepsis • intravenous access • intravenous continuous infusion • intravenous intermittent infusion.

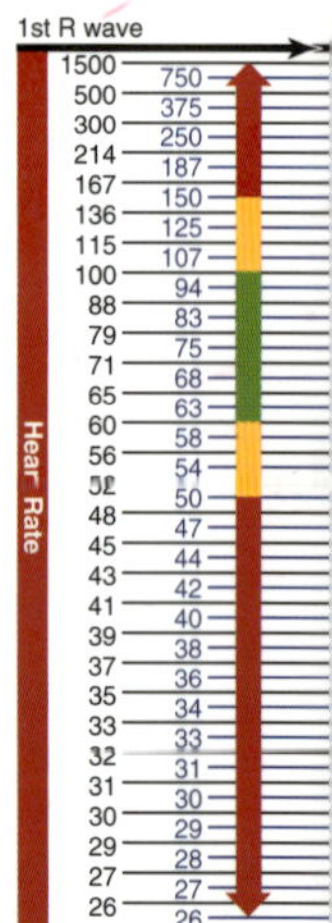

Look for our other Davis's Notes titles
OB/GYN & Peds Notes • Physical Assessment
Check-Off Notes • MedSurg Notes • NCLEX-RN® Notes

Beginning Point

Measurement

0.04	0.08
0.12	0.16
0.20	0.24
0.28	0.32
0.36	0.40
0.44	0.48
0.52	0.56
0.60	0.64
0.68	0.72
0.76	

Visit us at www.FADavis.com
F.A. Davis Company •
Independent Publishers Since 1879

ISBN: 978-0-8036-4024-5

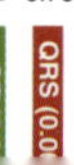

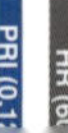

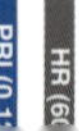

QRS (0.0